# Fit for Two

## The Official YMCA Prenatal Exercise Guide

*YMCA of the USA*
*with*
*Thomas W. Hanlon*

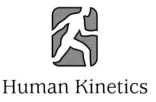

Human Kinetics

## Library of Congress Cataloging-in-Publication Data

Fit for two : the official YMCA prenatal exercise guide / YMCA of the
    USA, with Thomas W. Hanlon.
        p.    cm.
    Includes bibliographical references and index.
    ISBN 0-87322-828-6
    1. Pregnancy. 2. Exercise for women. 3. Relaxation. I. Hanlon,
    Thomas W.   II. YMCA of the USA.
    RG558.7.F56   1995
    618.2'4--dc20                                                          94-44684
                                                                              CIP

ISBN: 0-87322-828-6

**Developmental Editor:** Mary E. Fowler; **Technical and Exercise Consultant:** Rebecca
Nef-Heffernan; **Assistant Editors:** Dawn Roselund, Erik Dafforn, and Henry Woolsey;
**Copyeditor:** Barbara Field; **Proofreader:** Anne Meyer Byler; **Indexer:** Barbara E.
Cohen; **Typesetters and Layout Artists:** Ruby Zimmerman, Kathy Boudreau-Fuoss,
and Stuart Cartwright; **Text Designer:** Stuart Cartwright; **Cover Designer:** Jack
Davis; **Photographer (cover):** Esbin-Anderson/Photo Network; **Photographers
(interior):** Wilmer Zehr and Karen Maier; **Illustrator:** Beth Young; **On the cover:**
Kelly Tyler; **Printer:** United Graphics

Human Kinetics books are available at special discounts for bulk purchase. Special
editions or book excerpts can also be created to specification. For details, contact the
Special Sales Manager at Human Kinetics.

The YMCA of the USA does not operate any prenatal exercise programs.

Printed in the United States of America      10   9   8   7   6   5   4   3

**Human Kinetics**
Web site: http://www.humankinetics.com/

*United States:* Human Kinetics, P.O. Box 5076, Champaign, IL 61825-5076
1-800-747-4457
e-mail: humank@hkusa.com

*Canada:* Human Kinetics, 475 Devonshire Road, Unit 100, Windsor, ON N8Y 2L5
1-800-465-7301 (in Canada only)
e-mail: humank@hkcanada.com

*Europe:* Human Kinetics, P.O. Box IW14, Leeds LS16 6TR, United Kingdom
(44) 1132 781708
e-mail: humank@hkeurope.com

*Australia:* Human Kinetics, 57A Price Avenue, Lower Mitcham, South Australia 5062
(088) 277 1555
e-mail: humank@hkaustralia.com

*New Zealand:* Human Kinetics, P.O. Box 105-231, Auckland 1
(09) 523 3462
e-mail: humank@hknewz.com

# Contents

# Preface

If you want to learn how to exercise smartly and safely during your pregnancy, *Fit for Two: The Official YMCA Prenatal Exercise Guide* is for you. Prenatal exercise classes are popular because women want to know what activities and exercises are safe and effective, what will help them feel better during their pregnancy, and what can speed their recovery from childbirth. This guide provides you all that—and offers you two exercise programs, one on land and one in water, that will help you maintain or even improve your health and fitness as you approach the birth of your child. (*Fit for Two* does not refer to exercising your baby after birth.)

Part I of *Fit for Two: The Official YMCA Prenatal Exercise Guide* shows you how to exercise safely and wisely during your pregnancy. Chapter 1 explains the benefits of prenatal exercise, describes the physiological changes that take place during pregnancy and how they affect exercise, and explores other factors that affect your fitness and health.

Chapter 2 examines healthy prenatal exercise goals and how to attain those goals by taking part in an exercise class or setting up your own program. It lays out the basic components of a healthy program and states what activities are safe, what are unsafe, and what are signs to stop exercising. It also includes information on conditions that restrict exercise and guidelines for walking, jogging, swimming, and strength training. Chapter 2 provides the revised prenatal and postpartum exercise guidelines established in 1994 by the American College of Obstetricians and Gynecologists (ACOG).

Part II contains two exercise programs—one for land, one for water—and a chapter on relaxation and breathing exercises. Chapter 3 provides help on constructing your own workout plan for a land aerobics program, and it shows and describes the exercises themselves. Chapter 4 offers the same information for an aquatic exercise program. And chapter 5 explores breathing exercises and relaxation techniques that will help you both during your pregnancy and during labor and delivery.

Although this guide is designed to be used in YMCA prenatal exercise classes, you can also use it to work out on your own. Either way, any exercise program you undertake during your pregnancy should first be approved by your medical caregiver. If you are using this guide in conjunction with a YMCA prenatal exercise class, you may be required to go through a participant screening process to ascertain whether your exercise should be restricted, closely monitored, or preempted. Although the majority of women can exercise during their pregnancy with no problems, certain conditions (which we discuss in chapter 2) make it unwise. So if you're working out on your own, get approval from your medical caregiver first.

The programs in *Fit for Two: The Official YMCA Prenatal Exercise Guide* are appropriate for regular exercisers as well as beginners. The exercises themselves will help women stretch and tone muscles, regardless of their fitness level; the intensity of the aerobic portion of the workout can be controlled by the individual. In general, however, intensity and competitiveness in working out are discouraged; controlled effort and gradual progression are encouraged.

The YMCA cares about all aspects of your health and well-being. This prenatal exercise program is one of many YMCA programs designed to help you

- **grow personally**. We encourage people to set personal goals and work toward them through programs structured to help develop healthy self-images.

- **clarify values**. Y programs provide opportunities for reflection on personal values and the relationship between stated values and actual behavior. We encourage values that reflect Christian traditions and beliefs.

- **improve personal and family relationships**. The YMCA helps people develop cooperative attitudes and communication skills through programs for individuals and families.

- **appreciate diversity**. Y programs encourage diversity of thought, cultures, religions, and ethnic traditions, leading to communication and understanding among all people.

- **become better leaders and supporters**. In YMCA programs, shared leadership and support are basic organizational principles that are taught, practiced, and encouraged.

- **develop specific skills**. The development of individual skills is essential in accomplishing personal goals and in improving confidence and self-esteem.

- **have fun**. Fun, enjoyment, and laughter are essential qualities of all programs and contribute to people feeling good about themselves and the YMCA.

Be safe, be smart, and enjoy the benefits of prenatal exercise!

# Acknowledgments

The YMCA of the USA would like to acknowledge the contributions of the following individuals to the YMCA Prenatal Exercise project, which included the development of *Fit for Two: The Official YMCA Prenatal Exercise Guide* and *The YMCA Prenatal Exercise Instructor Guide.* Mike Spezzano and Lynne Vaughan of the YMCA of the USA provided staff leadership for the project. Tom Massey coordinated the project and the development of both resources.

The following YMCA staff served as the primary review team for the project:

| | |
|---|---|
| Luann Champlin | Mt. Madonna YMCA, Morgan Hill, CA |
| Michele Collins | Westerly-Pawcatuck YMCA, Westerly, RI |
| Jan Gross-Brucato | Limestone YMCA, Maysville, KY |
| Judi Gladieux | Eastern Toledo YMCA, Oregon, OH |
| Cheryl Houghtelin | Knoxville YMCA, Knoxville, TN |
| Brenda Jurich | Spokane YMCA, Spokane, WA |
| Cindy Koenig | Countryside-Warren YMCA, Lebanon, OH |
| Mary Treadaway | Southwest Milwaukee YMCA, Greenfield, WI |

The following YMCA staff reviewed the exercises:

| | |
|---|---|
| Joanne Bullock | Rockford YMCA, Rockford, IL |
| Kathi Cook | Chicago, IL |
| Barbara Norby-Muller | New City YMCA, Chicago, IL |
| Laura Slane | YMCA of the USA |
| Mary Treadaway | Southwest Milwaukee YMCA, Greenfield, WI |

Thanks also to Rebecca Nef-Heffernan, technical and exercise consultant.

# EXERCISING SAFELY DURING PREGNANCY

"Can I still exercise now that I'm pregnant?"

"I haven't been exercising before—but now that I'm pregnant I want to start an exercise program. Is that okay?"

"What activities are safe—and what are unsafe?"

"How much can I do?"

These are typical questions women ask about exercise once they become pregnant. In Part I we answer these and similar questions. For women without medical complications, prenatal exercise can be not only safe but beneficial—even for those who have been sedentary.

Chapter 1 explores the benefits of prenatal exercise and helps you understand the physiological changes taking place and how those changes affect your exercise. Chapter 2 helps you sort out what activities are safe and what are unsafe, indicates what conditions would restrict exercise, and provides guidelines for specific activities and for prenatal exercise in general.

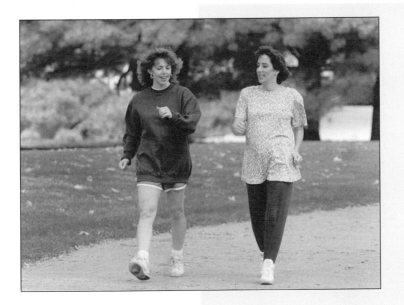

# Chapter 1

# Exercise, Health, and Pregnancy

**E**xercising during a pregnancy used to be taboo. Women were told to stay off their feet as much as possible; a sedentary lifestyle was encouraged. Now, however, the medical profession generally agrees that moderate exercise is safe for women who have no medical complications or preexisting conditions, such as vaginal bleeding or a history of miscarriages. (Risks and warning signs are explored in more detail in chapter 2.)

If you are cleared by your medical caregiver to participate in an exercise program, rest assured that exercising during your pregnancy can be both safe and beneficial. Let's look at ways prenatal exercise can help you.

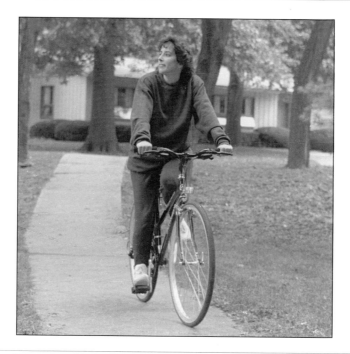

Increased stamina can help during labor and strengthens the muscles most affected by pregnancy: the pelvic floor muscles, abdominals, and lower back muscles.

## BENEFITS OF EXERCISE

Exercising won't necessarily make your labor easier—but it will help in many ways. Barbara Holstein, in *Shaping Up for a Healthy Pregnancy*, cites these prenatal exercise benefits:

- Improved circulation
- Enhanced muscular balance
- Reduced swelling
- Eased gastrointestinal discomforts, including constipation
- Reduced leg cramps
- Strengthened abdominal muscles
- Eased postpartum recovery

Many common discomforts of pregnancy—including varicose veins, backaches, and muscle and joint soreness—can be alleviated by exercise. Women can increase their stamina, which will help them while in labor, and they can strengthen and tone the muscles affected most by pregnancy: the pelvic floor muscles, abdominals, and lower back muscles.

A good prenatal exercise program can also improve posture—which is adversely affected by the growing uterus and expanding abdomen, which cause the pelvis to tilt forward. Exercises to strengthen the buttocks, back, shoulder, and stomach muscles help keep the body in alignment and decrease the discomfort associated with unhealthy posture.

---

### MORE EXERCISE, HEALTHIER BABIES?

In 1993, *American Health* reported on a 2-year study conducted in New York that showed women who work out for 30 min, 5 days a week, have bigger, healthier babies. Women who burned 1,000 calories a week delivered babies who weighed about 5% more than those delivered by sedentary mothers. Pregnant women who burned 2,000 calories a week gave birth to babies who weighed 10% more than babies born to inactive women.

---

A 1989 study appearing in the *American Journal of Obstetrics and Gynecology* showed that women who exercised moderately and regularly during the last trimester perceived their labor as less painful than women who did not exercise. This could be due in part to the increased level of endorphins in the bodies of the exercisers; endorphins act as a natural pain reliever.

Finally, prenatal exercise can enhance your sense of well-being, control, and body image. It can help you become comfortable with your body as your baby grows within your womb. Next we'll look at the changes your body undergoes—and how those changes affect your exercise.

## BODY CHANGES AND EXERCISE IMPLICATIONS

Your body undergoes many changes during pregnancy—for instance, your uterus grows to about 1,000 times its normal size! Your uterus pushes on your diaphragm, which can alter your breathing. Your heart enlarges, your veins become softer to allow for increased

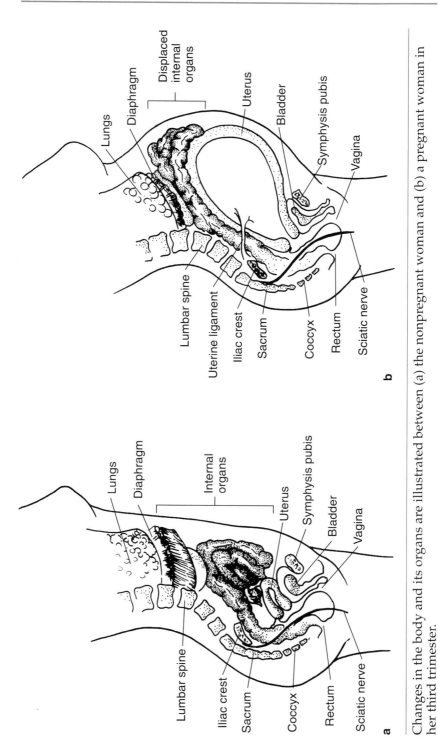

Changes in the body and its organs are illustrated between (a) the nonpregnant woman and (b) a pregnant woman in her third trimester.

blood flow, your ligaments loosen, and your breasts enlarge. These are just a few ways your body prepares for childbirth. Some of the major changes that take place within your body, along with their implications for exercise, follow.

## BREATHING CHANGES

The diaphragm is a muscle that separates the lungs from the abdominal cavity and that aids in breathing. The expanding uterus presses on and moves the diaphragm upward, making it difficult to draw the diaphragm down far enough when you inhale. As a result, you may feel breathless, especially if you are exercising vigorously. You may also hyperventilate (breathe quickly and not inhale deeply enough), causing lightheadedness or dizziness.

To compensate for the restricted diaphragm, the rib cage flares out to allow adequate room for the lungs. Oxygen consumption actually increases by 15% to 20% during pregnancy, although the oxygen reserve—the extra oxygen that's stored in your blood and muscles—decreases. (This reserve is used when the body needs more oxygen; because a pregnant woman's body supplies oxygen for both herself and her baby, that reserve supply is tapped into.) Increased progesterone levels raise the normal breathing rate by 45%. Exercising can increase your aerobic capacity during pregnancy; if you don't exercise it will likely decrease.

### Exercise Implications

- Watch your exercise intensity; don't overexert. Overexertion can contribute to breathlessness and hyperventilation. To avoid hyperventilation, breathe slowly and evenly, inhaling and exhaling deeply.
- Don't hold your breath. Many women have a tendency to do so during exertion; this is called the Valsalva maneuver. It can cause dizziness or fainting.
- Lift your arms up and out to ease breathing. This relieves the pressure the uterus puts on the diaphragm and allows the rib cage to expand.
- If you get stitches, cramps that occur in the rib cage muscles, massage the sore muscles, blow out forcefully, and lift your knees.

- Exercise in low humidity to lessen the chances of getting nose-bleeds or nasal stuffiness due to nasal passage swelling.

## HEART AND CIRCULATORY CHANGES

During pregnancy, the heart wall thickens and the heart enlarges and moves upward because of pressure from the diaphragm. Blood volume increases by 30% to 50%; your resting heart rate may increase by up to 20%. Cardiac output (the amount of blood pumped by the heart) increases by 40% to 50% to meet the needs of your growing uterus and baby. Yet your cardiac reserve (the capacity of the heart to meet the body's demands) diminishes. This means that you'll get tired sooner, especially during rigorous exercise, because of the increased oxygen requirements—for both you and your baby—and the increased work of breathing as your enlarged uterus presses on your diaphragm.

Strenuous exertion can cause an irregular or excessively pounding heartbeat; if this happens, you should stop exercising.

Blood vessels soften and stretch to accommodate the increase in blood volume. This stretching can result in varicose veins, hemor-rhoids, and swelling. These are most common in the second and third trimesters.

In some cases the vessels don't stretch; instead they constrict and cause blood pressure to rise. If this rise occurs during pregnancy it is known as pregnancy-induced hypertension—a serious and poten-tially fatal disease. Symptoms include fluid retention, sudden swell-ing, blurred vision, and severe headaches. You should have your blood pressure checked regularly throughout your pregnancy.

Exercise increases both blood pressure and pulse; these increases can remain for 15 min after exercises.

### Exercise Implications

- Exercise comfortably, not intensely.
- Don't exercise to exhaustion; stop exercising when you become fatigued.
- If your heartbeat is irregular or pounds excessively, stop exercis-ing. Walk for a few minutes and then rest until your heart rate returns to normal. While resting, make sure to hold your head higher than your heart.

- Exercise can help ease varicose veins because it increases circulation.
- Rise and change directions slowly to avoid dizziness.

## STOMACH AND INTESTINAL CHANGES

Hormonal changes cause activity in the stomach and intestines to slow down. The stomach and intestines are moved upward by the enlarged uterus; this can cause heartburn and indigestion. Constipation is a problem for about half of all pregnant women because of the slowed digestive process. Nausea and vomiting—commonly known as "morning sickness"—often occur, usually during the first 3 months, because of hormonal changes. The nausea is more severe with an empty stomach. Excessive vomiting can cause dehydration.

### Exercise Implications

- Eat a healthy snack an hour or so before exercise—a piece of fruit or some crackers.
- To lessen the effects of nausea, don't let your stomach get empty. Eat a peeled apple, a few crackers, or dry toast an hour or so before exercising, and slow down your exercise.
- Exercise at the same time each day.
- Drink enough fluids—six to eight glasses per day. Be especially careful to drink enough fluids if you're vomiting.

## KIDNEY AND BLADDER CHANGES

The growing uterus presses on the bladder, causing you to feel the need to urinate more frequently (especially early on and late in the pregnancy). This doesn't mean there's a problem, and you shouldn't drink less to compensate. Many women tend to leak urine late in their pregnancy. Fluids are often retained late in the pregnancy; swelling of the legs and ankles is common, but swelling in the hands and face may indicate a problem that should be checked out by your caregiver. Exercise can help reduce swelling by increasing circulation. When not exercising, elevating your legs and wearing support hose can help. However, avoid clothing that binds tightly in one place.

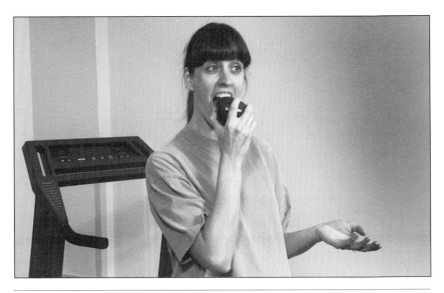

To lessen the effects of nausea, don't let your stomach get empty. Eat a peeled apple, crackers, or dry toast about an hour before exercising, and slow down your exercise.

### Exercise Implications

- Doing pelvic floor exercises can help control the bladder muscles and prevent leaking urine.
- Make sure there is a bathroom nearby for frequent stops! You may also want to wear a minipad.

## MUSCULAR, JOINT, AND POSTURAL CHANGES

Your uterus grows and presses on your pelvic area during the second trimester; coupled with your weight gain, this causes your center of gravity to shift. The hormone relaxin causes your ligaments to relax and your joints to soften and stretch (leaving you prone to joint injury in the third trimester). The hip joints, in particular, become sore.

The stomach muscles can become strained as they stretch, and the lower back, whose muscles tighten, can become sore. Many women experience a mild separation of the abdominal muscles; this condition is called *diastasis recti* (see page 15 for how to check for this). Diastasis recti is not serious, but its presence will affect your workout.

Lordosis, or swayback, is common in pregnancy. It can be caused by shifting of the center of gravity, which moves forward in relation to the spinal column, and by the weight of the uterus on the pelvic area. As the pelvis tilts forward, the lumbar curve in the lower back is accentuated. The shoulders often slump forward to counterbalance the exaggerated curving of the lower back. Poor posture can cause backaches and muscle spasms.

## Exercise Implications

- Make directional changes slowly and avoid complicated foot patterns as your center of gravity shifts.
- Don't stretch to your maximum, and be careful about making sudden changes in direction as your joints loosen.
- Check regularly to see if your abdominal muscles are separating, and modify your abdominal exercises if necessary (see page 14).
- Strengthen your abdominals, your back muscles, and your buttocks to help achieve a healthy posture.

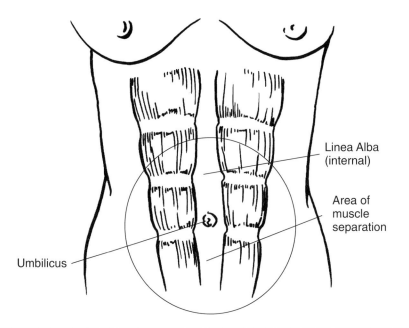

Separation of the abdominal muscles (diastasis recti) often occurs during pregnancy.

---

### SUPINE HYPOTENSIVE SYNDROME

When the enlarged uterus places pressure on the inferior vena cava (the vein that returns blood to the heart from the torso and legs), nausea, dizziness, breathing difficulties, and a claustrophobic feeling can occur. This condition, called *supine hypotensive syndrome*, is brought on most often by lying on your back after your first trimester of pregnancy. It is the major reason the American College of Obstetricians and Gynecologists advises pregnant women not to perform exercises while lying on their back after their first trimester.

If you are lying on your back and feel any of the symptoms mentioned, simply roll onto your left side until you feel better.

---

## HORMONAL CHANGES

Several hormonal changes take place, helping to regulate your pregnancy and promote growth:

- *Estrogen* levels rise, stimulating growth of the uterus and breasts. High levels of estrogen can cause you to retain water; the increase in this hormone can also cause nausea (especially during the first trimester) and joint looseness.

- *Progesterone* levels also rise, helping the uterine walls thicken and develop and inhibiting smooth muscle contraction (thus relaxing the uterus and keeping it from contracting excessively). Progesterone also helps maintain a healthy blood pressure by relaxing and dilating the walls of the blood vessels, allowing for the greater blood volume. It also relaxes the stomach and intestines, promoting greater absorption of nutrients. The core body temperature is raised by progesterone, which affects the hypothalamus, the body's thermostat. The increase in progesterone causes many women to feel fatigued.

- *Relaxin* softens ligaments, cartilage, and the cervix, allowing these tissues to spread during delivery. It also inhibits uterine activity.

- *Insulin* levels increase during pregnancy; 1 out of 300 women contract gestational diabetes mellitus. The extent to which exercise is affected depends on the severity of the condition. Symptoms of diabetes mellitus include constant thirst and excessive urination. This condition often disappears after pregnancy.

Diabetes can greatly affect the health of your baby. If you were diabetic before your pregnancy, or you acquire gestational diabetes, you should have your blood glucose levels checked and your exercise participation monitored by your medical caregiver. Exercise can help you control your diabetes by increasing your maximum oxygen uptake, decreasing your blood pressure, and helping control your glucose levels.

### Exercise Implications

- Pay attention to the warning signs of diabetes mellitus: excessive urination and thirst. If you have diabetes, have your glucose levels checked frequently and your exercise participation monitored by your caregiver.
- Wear clothing that helps you keep cool during workouts.
- Don't stretch to your maximum; as your ligaments become softer and looser, you can injure yourself this way.

## BREAST CHANGES

The breasts enlarge and can become sensitive; the nipples and areolas (the dark skin around the nipples) grow and become darker. Breast growth continues throughout the first trimester; veins may become more prominent. Colostrum, a mixture of water, protein, minerals, and antibodies that the baby will feed on for the first few days, usually develops in the mother's breasts by 12 to 14 weeks. Not all women develop colostrum; it's not a concern if you don't.

### Exercise Implications

- Wear a supportive, comfortable sport bra when you exercise.

## PELVIC FLOOR CHANGES

The pelvic floor muscles act as a sling to support the abdominal and pelvic organs, forming a figure eight around the urethra, vagina, and anus. During birth, the pelvic floor muscles stretch to allow the baby to come out. When these muscles are toned and strong, they aid in having a controlled birth. Because of the weight of the uterus, they can sag during pregnancy. Strong pelvic floor muscles also alleviate the common prenatal problem of leaking urine, because these muscles control the bladder.

### Exercise Implications

- Pelvic floor (Kegel) exercises are extremely important in toning and maintaining these muscles. These exercises can be done at any time in any place. Do a total of 50 repetitions daily of the various pelvic floor exercises shown in chapter 3.

## SEPARATION OF THE ABDOMINAL MUSCLES

As mentioned earlier the stomach, or rectus, muscles can separate down the center of the abdomen, a condition called diastasis recti. This condition can be caused by the baby pushing on the uterine wall, hormonal changes, or straining of the muscles. This condition occurs most commonly in the second trimester. It is not painful, and you can continue to exercise when your stomach muscles separate, but you may need to adjust your abdominal exercise if the separation is greater than an inch.

### Exercise Implications

- Do the self-test for diastasis recti frequently; it's best to check before every exercise session (see "Self-Test for Abdominal Muscle Separation" on page 15).

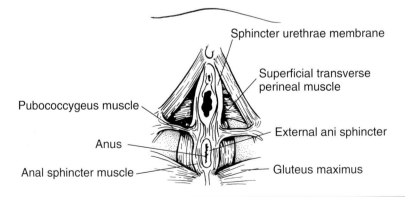

The pelvic floor muscles support and encircle the urethra, vagina, and anus.

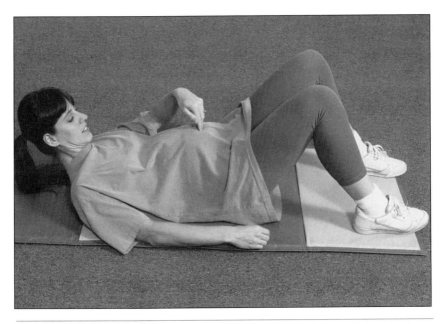

Check before every exercise session for separation of your abdominal muscles. If the separation is greater than 1 in. wide, you'll need to adjust your abdominal exercise.

- Check with your exercise instructor or your medical caregiver for exercise modifications if your muscle separation is greater than 1 in. One exercise that helps strengthen separated abdominals is modified curl-ups (page 53).

### SELF-TEST FOR ABDOMINAL MUSCLE SEPARATION

Lie on your back with your knees bent and your feet flat on the floor. Place your fingertips just above or below your navel. Lift your head and shoulders off the floor and pull your chin to your chest. Press firmly on your stomach, feeling for any separation between the bands of vertical muscles. If the separation is greater than two fingers' width, you should be careful not to strain your abdominal muscles as you exercise. Ask your medical caregiver or exercise instructor how you should modify your exercise. The modified curl-up exercise on page 53 helps strengthen abdominal muscles that have separated.

# FACTORS AFFECTING FITNESS AND HEALTH

Your health and fitness are affected by many factors before, during, and after your pregnancy. In the following pages, we'll look at some of these factors, especially as they relate to your fitness and health during pregnancy. Questions regarding these or any other health-related issues should be taken up with your medical caregiver.

## NUTRITION

Nutritional needs increase during pregnancy; however, if you were eating a healthy diet before, the adjustments should be easy. You'll need to ingest about 300 more calories a day (or a little more if you're exercising regularly). These calories should be high in protein, calcium, and iron. Iron-rich foods include liver and other organ meats; red meat; egg yolks; prune and apple juices; and peas, beans, lentils, oysters, almonds, and walnuts.

Your calcium needs increase to 1,200 mg a day, equivalent to a quart of skim or lowfat milk. If you're allergic to milk, you can get your calcium through Lactaid or acidophilus milk; other calcium-rich include yogurt, buttermilk, cheese, and pudding.

You'll also need to increase your intake of folic acid, which helps cells grow. Folic acid is found in liver; green, leafy vegetables; and yeast. Your medical caregiver may prescribe supplements if you are low in iron and folic acid, but you should also increase your intake of these nutrients through foods.

As always, you'll want to maintain a balanced diet, eating fresh fruits and vegetables, whole grains and cereals, dairy products, protein foods, and drinking six to eight cups of liquids per day. It's better to eat five or six small meals a day rather than two or three large ones, because the large ones may cause nausea. The USDA has set general guidelines for daily nutrition for each of the five food groups.

Nausea and vomiting, which occur most often during the first 3 months, can keep you from meeting your nutritional needs. You may need to supplement your diet, but any supplement should be prescribed by your medical caregiver. If you're nauseated, you'll feel better by keeping something in your stomach, such as dry toast or a peeled apple.

You can eat a vegetarian diet while you're pregnant, but you'll need to drink milk to gain all the nutrients you need. Consult your medical caregiver regarding your diet if you're a vegetarian.

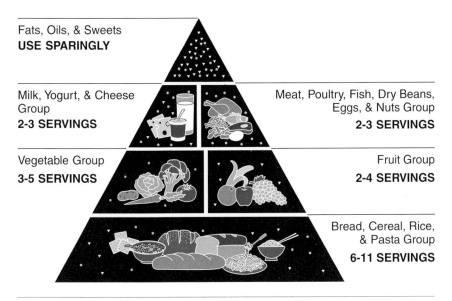

The USDA food pyramid shows a recommended daily diet. Ask your caregiver how to adjust this diet during your pregnancy.

Source: U.S. Department of Agriculture/U.S. Department of Health and Human Services.

## CAFFEINE

Caffeine causes calcium to be excreted through urination, reducing the amount of this vital nutrient available to both you and your baby. When you are pregnant, caffeine is eliminated more slowly from your body, thereby increasing its effects on you and your baby. Caffeine increases the production of adrenaline hormones, which cause a temporary decrease in the oxygen and nutrients available to your baby.

A study reported in the *Journal of the American Medical Association* showed that pregnant women who drank one to three cups of caffeinated coffee a day doubled their chances of miscarriage—and women who drank more than three cups a day tripled their risks. Even drinking three cups a day the month *before* conception doubled the risk of miscarriage. No studies have shown caffeine to be linked to birth defects, low birth weight, or any congenital problems.

To be safe, either stop ingesting caffeine while you're trying to conceive and during your pregnancy or keep your intake under 300 mg per day. See the following chart to help you calculate caffeine levels.

**The Caffeine Count.**   Caffeine levels vary widely, depending on the product and how it has been prepared, but this chart will give you an idea of the amount of caffeine found in certain products:

| Product | Caffeine (mg) |
| --- | --- |
| Coffee, drip or brewed, 6 oz | 80 to 175 |
| Coffee, instant, 6 oz | 60 to 100 |
| Coffee, decaffeinated, 6 oz | 2 to 5 |
| Tea, 5-min steep, 6 oz | 20 to 100 |
| Hot cocoa, 6 oz | 2 to 20 |
| Coca-Cola, 12 oz | 30 to 45 |
| Milk chocolate, 1 oz | 1 to 10 |
| Bittersweet chocolate, 1 oz | 5 to 35 |
| Chocolate cake, 1 slice | 20 to 30 |
| Anacin, Empirin, or Midol, 2 pills | 64 |
| Excedrin, 2 pills | 130 |
| NoDoz, 2 pills | 200 |

## TOBACCO

Lung cancer has surpassed breast cancer as the leading killer of women. About 28% of women smoke, and smoking poses as great or even greater danger for your fetus because, with each inhalation, your womb fills with toxins that inhibit nutrient and oxygen delivery and expose your unborn child to cancer-causing agents.

Smokers are twice as likely to have babies who weigh less than 5.2 lb. It has been shown that the more you smoke, the less your baby weighs—and with this lighter weight come all sorts of problems. Smokers run greater risks of having babies with higher rates of brain damage, cerebral palsy, lowered IQ, learning and behavioral disabilities, and perinatal death (death that occurs around the time of birth). Women who smoke have an increased chance of having premature babies. The incidence of Sudden Infant Death Syndrome (SIDS) is 50% higher for babies of mothers who smoke.

If that's not enough, smokers are more likely to have ectopic pregnancies (where babies are born in unusual positions), vaginal bleeding, miscarriages, and stillbirths.

Passive smoking—inhaling someone else's smoke—is also a hazard to the health of both you and your fetus.

If you smoke and you can't quit, don't despair. Even cutting down helps. The most damage is done in the last 4 months. Women who stop smoking during their pregnancy generally have the same size babies as women who never smoked.

For help with quitting, call your local office of the American Cancer Society, the American Heart Association, the American Lung Association, or a hospital.

## ALCOHOL

Alcohol is similar to tobacco in that it can cause great damage to the fetus—and that stopping or cutting back at any point is helpful.

Alcohol interferes with the absorption of nutrients by the baby. The same level of alcohol that enters the mother's bloodstream also enters that of the fetus. Thus, the more you drink the more harm you can do to your baby. It is best not to drink at all during your pregnancy, or to drink *very* rarely and minimally (such as one drink on a special occasion).

As little as two drinks a day, or an occasional heavy binge, have been associated with Fetal Alcohol Syndrome (FAS), which results in disabilities ranging from mental retardation to physical disability; facial malformation; central nervous system disorders; and bone, heart, and urogenital problems. Six thousand babies are born with FAS each year.

Drinking early in pregnancy is more likely to result in birth defects; drinking late in pregnancy can cause low birth weight. Even one or two drinks twice a week can increase the risk of spontaneous abortion and learning impairment. There is no known safe quantity to drink.

The U.S. Surgeon General has stated, "Women should avoid all alcoholic beverages during pregnancy because of their risk to birth defects."

## MEDICATIONS AND DRUGS

All use of medications and drugs—including pain relievers, tranquilizers, antihistamines, and antiemetics (which control nausea and vomiting)—should be cleared with your medical caregiver.

Even aspirin can be harmful to the fetus because it is an anticoagulant, which means that if you get cut, for instance, you will bleed longer after you use it. Aspirin can also rob the fetus of oxygen and postpone the onset of labor.

Illicit drugs are even more dangerous. Cocaine users have a 25% higher chance of a preterm delivery. Pregnant women who use cocaine are more prone to heart attacks and more likely to have babies with low birth weight, smaller heads and brains, fragile nervous systems, and a range of long-lasting physical, emotional, and behavioral problems.

Women who smoke marijuana two to five times a week are more likely to have premature babies. Drugs such as heroin, methadone, and PCP (angel dust) are addictive to the baby as well as the mother.

Crack, a form of cocaine, is associated with miscarriages, reduced birth weight, stillbirth, malformation, and SIDS. Crack can also cause deformed hearts, lungs, and digestive systems, as well as brain hemorrhages and strokes.

According to the National Institute on Drug Abuse, 5 million women of childbearing age used illicit drugs in 1988. About 10% of babies born each year—or about 375,000—are born with some illicit drug in their blood. The cost for treating a drug-addicted newborn can be as high as $200,000.

## SAUNAS AND HOT TUBS

The extreme heat from saunas, hot tubs, and whirlpools can be dangerous to you and your baby, especially in the first half of your pregnancy. As your body temperature rises, the development of your fetus can be impeded. Repeatedly raising your body temperature for long periods can cause birth defects or even fetal death.

It's probably safe in the second half of your pregnancy to take a sauna or soak in a hot tub, but it's best to monitor your temperature and not let it rise more than a degree before you step out to cool down. Do this by taking your oral temperature before you step in and also while you're in the sauna or hot tub. Keeping your shoulders and arms out of the water will help keep you cooler.

## RELAXATION AND BREATHING TECHNIQUES

Knowing how to relax both throughout your pregnancy and during labor can be a great help to you. The relaxation and breathing techniques presented in chapter 5 will help you relax and control your pain during delivery. They will help you feel comfortable, calm, and in control. These techniques can also help you release muscular and mental tension, conserve energy, and reduce stress.

## RADIATION

In large doses, X-rays, which contain ionizing radiation, can harm your fetus. X-rays are used to diagnose internal organ problems. You shouldn't work in areas—such as dental and medical offices—where radiation levels are high; prolonged exposure can be harmful. Ultrasound is now commonly used in place of X-rays to study the fetus. You should request ultrasound if your physician suggests using X-rays, and if possible, avoid having X-rays taken by your dentist.

It is unlikely that computer or video display terminals present much of a hazard to your fetus, although one study in the early 1980s linked miscarriages with women who worked at a VDT for more than 20 hr a week. However, more recent studies have not shown any such link.

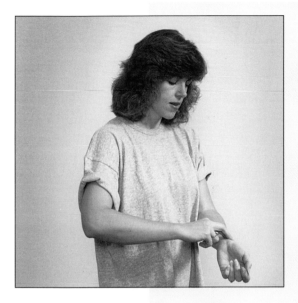

# Chapter 2

# Exercise Goals and Guidelines

You've learned how prenatal exercise can help you, how your changing body affects how you approach exercise, and how a variety of factors can positively and negatively affect your and your baby's health. In this chapter, we'll explore safe and effective ways to exercise, but first we'll look at healthy exercise goals—and how those goals differ from those of a woman who is not pregnant.

# HEALTHY EXERCISE GOALS

Maybe you've been sedentary in recent years and are prompted to work out by your pregnancy. Perhaps you're a weekend athlete, playing an occasional game of tennis, or you might walk or swim a few times a week. Or maybe you're a veteran triathlete and have trained seriously for years. Regardless of your exercise and fitness background, as you enter your pregnancy, you should have specific goals in mind—and prenatal exercise goals differ in significant ways from exercise goals in general.

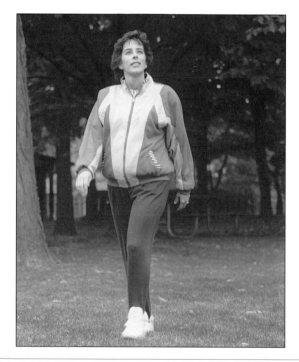

Walking can help maintain cardiovascular fitness and tone muscles. Many call walking the ideal exercise for pregnant women.

According to fitness expert Kenneth Cooper, general exercise objectives women have are to

- improve cardiovascular fitness,
- lose weight,
- build or shape the body, and
- have fun.

Two of those four objectives—improving cardiovascular fitness and having fun—are appropriate for prenatal exercise, but obviously losing weight and body shaping are not! According to prenatal exercise expert Barbara Holstein, pregnant women can work safely to

- maintain muscular strength,
- improve or maintain cardiovascular fitness,
- improve flexibility,
- improve posture, and
- have fun.

In 1985, the American College of Obstetricians and Gynecologists (ACOG) stated that "the goals of exercise during pregnancy and the postpartum period should be to maintain the highest level of fitness consistent with maximum safety."

Those goals are important to keep in mind as you exercise during your pregnancy—regardless of your exercise history. But depending on your fitness level and exercise background, you may wonder how those goals will affect your approach to exercise.

## WHAT IF I'VE BEEN SEDENTARY?

Assuming you have no conditions that would restrict your exercise (see p. 34), you can safely begin an exercise program while you're pregnant. It's best to begin a program at the beginning of the second trimester because the possibility of overheating is more serious during the first trimester. Start easy and progress slowly. Walking, swimming, and stationary biking are good activities to complement the exercises in this book. Of course, you should have any prenatal exercise program approved by your medical caregiver first (as should all women).

## WHAT IF I'M ALREADY MODERATELY WORKING OUT?

Chances are good that you can continue your workouts with little variation; you'll simply need to keep the prenatal exercise goals in mind and structure your workouts to keep within the guidelines established by the ACOG (see p. 30). You may have to adjust your activities or your intensity. Later in this chapter we discuss activities that are safe and unsafe.

## WHAT IF I'M A COMPETITIVE ATHLETE?

You may need to tone down your intensity. The ACOG guidelines were established to protect you and your fetus. Competition and intensity are out; controlled effort, comfort, and consistency are in. Remember, you're exercising now for the health benefits and to maintain fitness, not to improve performance. Use the talk test as well as pulse checks to monitor your exertion level. If you can talk comfortably while you're exercising, your intensity is okay. If not, slow down.

# EXERCISE PROGRAM COMPONENTS

The exercise program we've devised to help you achieve healthy exercise goals includes the following components.

## WARM-UP

The warm-up is essential to preparing muscles to work and stretch without being injured. Walking or leisurely riding a stationary bike are good ways to warm up, as is swimming slowly. The warm-up increases your heart rate, breathing, and blood flow and raises your body temperature. Even if you have a limited time to work out, don't shortcut your warm-up. Spend at least 5 min preparing your body for the workout.

## AEROBIC ACTIVITY

Aerobic activity—what many consider the "meat" of the workout—increases your heart rate and your maximum oxygen uptake, tones your muscles, and helps you maintain or even improve your fitness during pregnancy. Because of your increased oxygen requirements and increased breathing work, you'll have less oxygen available for aerobic exercise, so you will have to modify your intensity. Don't work out to exhaustion; stop when you get fatigued. Walking, swimming, and jogging are common and safe aerobic activities; other safe activities are discussed on page 36.

## STRENGTHENING EXERCISES

Exercises that strengthen your muscles help build tone and endurance. We have included exercises in this book that will help you strengthen all major body parts, including the abdominals, the shoulders and arms, the back, the legs, and the pelvic floor muscles. We suggest you strengthen all the major muscles of your body by doing the strengthening exercises in chapters 3 and 4.

## COOLDOWN

Cooling down helps your breathing and heart rate return to normal and inhibits blood, which has been pumping to your working muscles, from pooling in your extremities. You should cool down for 5 min at the end of your aerobic activity by simply decreasing the intensity of your activity or by walking. After your strengthening exercises, we recommend that you cool down with a few leisurely stretching exercises, holding the stretch for longer than normal and concentrating on deep breathing.

## STRETCHING EXERCISES

Stretching your muscles will lengthen them and increase their flexibility. During pregnancy, it is especially important to stretch slowly and gently because your joints are loosened by the increase in the hormones progesterone and relaxin. Don't stretch to your point of maximum resistance or use jerky, bouncy movements. Also, avoid stretches where your joints are unsupported because they can lead to injury. We suggest that you stretch for at least 5 min using the stretching exercises found in chapters 3 and 4.

## RELAXATION

Relaxation techniques can help you during both your pregnancy and your delivery. Through a variety of techniques, you can re-

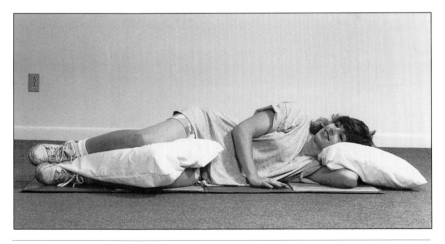

Relaxation techniques can release muscular tension and help you feel more comfortable, calm, and in control.

lease muscular and mental tension and feel more comfortable, calm, and in control. You'll find relaxation and breathing exercises in chapter 5.

# BODY AREAS EXERCISED

Our prenatal exercise program works all your major muscles and body areas, paying special attention to the areas most affected by pregnancy.

## ABDOMINALS

As the size of the uterus increases, the abdominal (stomach) muscles stretch. When a muscle is stretched for a prolonged period—such as during pregnancy—it tends to weaken. Yet the abdominal muscles need to be in good shape to support the increasing weight of the baby. That's why it's important to strengthen the abdominals.

As mentioned in chapter 1, the abdominal muscles can separate during pregnancy; this common and painless condition, called diastasis recti, occurs most often during the second trimester. Although not a serious condition, it does affect how you approach abdominal exercises. For more information on diastasis recti and how to check for it, see page 15.

## ARMS AND UPPER BODY

You'll use your arms, shoulders, and upper back muscles to lift, hold, and carry your baby, so it's important to strengthen these areas and to relieve tension in your shoulders and upper back.

## BACK

With the increasing weight of your baby in front, greater stress is placed on your back. Lower back pain is one of the most common discomforts of pregnancy. A strong back is vital to maintaining healthy posture; it's easy to develop lordosis, or exaggerated curvature of the spine, during pregnancy if your back is weak. Our exercises will help you tone and strengthen your back muscles to relieve discomfort and maintain healthy posture.

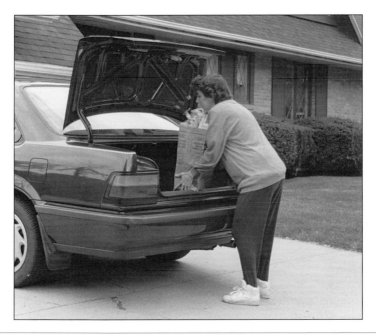

Lower back pain is common in pregnancy. It's vital to keep your back strong and maintain healthy posture.

## HEAD AND NECK

The neck and head can become tense and rigid, due in part to a shift in your center of gravity that can cause your shoulders to slump forward. Exercises to stretch the neck muscles will help ease tension in the neck and shoulders. Keep your jaw and face relaxed while performing exercises for the head and neck.

## LEGS AND LOWER EXTREMITIES

As your weight increases, your legs must support and carry a larger load. Swelling and varicose veins often occur in the legs; exercise can help reduce both conditions by increasing circulation.

## PELVIC FLOOR

The pelvic floor muscles—which act as a sling or hammock to support your uterus, bladder, bowel, and other pelvic organs—are of vital importance both during your pregnancy and throughout your life. The weight of the growing uterus can cause these muscles to sag; strengthening them can help you have a slow, controlled delivery. With weak pelvic floor muscles, the baby can come too quickly and cause the perineum muscles, directly below the pelvic floor, to tear.

Pelvic floor contractions can be performed at any time in any position, even in conjunction with other exercises. As you're doing arm circles, for example, you can also do pelvic floor exercises, which are described in chapters 3 and 4.

# EXERCISE GUIDELINES

The following guidelines are from exercise recommendations established by the ACOG in 1992 and 1994. The recommendations are paraphrased and commented upon.

- **Exercise at least three times per week.** Exercising less usually produces little or no cardiovascular improvement. Sporadic exercise is also harder to stick with; keeping a routine of at least three times per week will help you maintain or improve your fitness. If you're in an exercise class that meets twice a week, make sure you exercise at least once more each week on your own.

- **Don't exercise on your back after the first trimester.** Exercising on your back may put pressure on your inferior vena cava, the vein that returns blood from the legs and torso to the heart. Pressure on this vein can cause hypotension (abnormally low blood pressure), resulting in feelings of dizziness, nausea, and shortness of breath. (See "Supine Hypotensive Syndrome" on p. 12.) For the same reason, you should also avoid standing motionless for long periods.

- **Modify your intensity; listen to your body.** Less oxygen is available for aerobic exercise during pregnancy because of increased oxygen requirements and breathing difficulties. Don't exercise to exhaustion; stop when you get fatigued. While no studies have shown that you need to lower your target heart range during pregnancy, you shouldn't exceed 75% of your maximum heart rate. This will reduce the possibility of overheating, a primary concern in pregnancy, especially in the first trimester (see page 32). Use this formula to find your target heart range: (220 – age) $\times$ 60% to 75% = target heart range.

So, if you are 30 years old, your target heart range would be 114 to 142 ($190 \times 0.60 = 114$; $190 \times 0.75 = 142$). If you're 20, your target heart range would be 120 to 150 beats/min. Measure your heart rate during peak activity. (See "Monitoring Your Heart Rate" on p. 32).

Another accurate way to measure your exertion is using the rate of perceived exertion (RPE), according to Raul Artal-Mittelmark, MD, one of the original authors of the ACOG guidelines (see Figure 2.1). Artal Mittelmark says an appropriate exertion rate for pregnant women is defined as "somewhat hard" on the RPE scale. If your exertion is more difficult than "somewhat hard," then back off.

The ACOG also recommends that for exercise routines that involve repeated foot impacts (such as aerobic routines), you limit your time to no more than 30 min, keeping within your target heart range and taking a day of rest between sessions.

| | |
|---|---|
| 6 | No exertion at all |
| 7 | Extremely light |
| 8 | |
| 9 | Very light |
| 10 | |
| 11 | Light |
| 12 | |
| 13 | Somewhat hard |
| 14 | |
| 15 | Hard (heavy) |
| 16 | |
| 17 | Very hard |
| 18 | |
| 19 | Extremely hard |
| 20 | Maximal exertion |

© Gunnar Borg 1985

**Figure 2.1**    Borg perceived exertion scale (1985). Borg scale from *An Introduction to Borg's RPE Scale* (p. 7) by G. Borg, 1985, Ithaca, NY: Mouvement Publications. Copyright 1985 by Gunnar Borg. Reprinted by permission.

### MONITORING YOUR HEART RATE

Using your fingertips, find your pulse in your radial artery along the thumb side of your wrist. Or, using a light touch, find your carotid artery (in your neck, alongside your Adam's apple). Don't use your thumb to take your pulse because you can feel a pulse in it, too, and you may miscount.

Once you've found your pulse, count the beats for 10 sec. Multiply that count by 6 to figure your beats per minute. Remember to take your pulse at the peak of your activity—and if you are exceeding the maximum of your target heart range or you feel fatigued, slow down.

- **Don't jeopardize your balance.** Your center of gravity shifts during pregnancy; you can feel awkward and off balance, especially in the third trimester. Sudden changes in direction and jumping can cause injuries.

- **Avoid activities with the potential for even mild abdominal trauma.** On page 37 we discuss what activities are unsafe.

- **Be careful not to overheat, especially in the first trimester.** As mentioned, overheating is a concern during pregnancy, as is dehydration. Your body core temperature shouldn't exceed 38 °C (100 °F). When you're pregnant, you're more likely to have trouble keeping your body temperature down; exercising vigorously in hot, humid weather or when you have a fever makes matters worse. Drink liquids before and after exercise and, if necessary, during your workout. In warm weather, work out in loose-fitting, cotton clothes that "breathe," and if you're exercising indoors, the room should be well ventilated.

- **Warm up and cool down every time you exercise.** Warming up stretches and prepares your muscles for exercise and gets your blood circulating; warm up for at least 5 min before you begin your activity. An adequate warm-up—walking, stationary biking, or doing whatever activity you're preparing for at a slower pace—will help prevent injuries.

  Cooling down helps your heart rate return to normal and prevents blood from pooling in your extremities. A cooldown of 5 to 10 min of walking and leisurely stretching helps you recover more quickly from exercise than simply stopping.

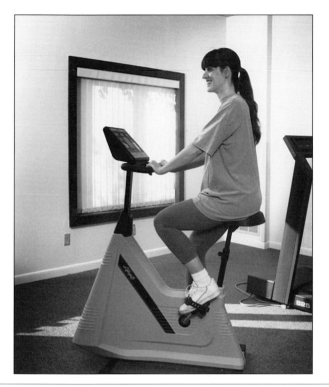

Warming up before a workout gets your blood circulating and prepares your muscles for exercise.

- **Exercise on a resilient floor.** If you're working out inside, a carpeted or wood floor helps reduce the shock to your feet and legs.
- **Don't flex your joints excessively or stretch to your limit.** Your joints are looser during pregnancy and more vulnerable to injury. This applies particularly to hip and knee joints. Also, avoid ballistic movements—jerky, bouncy motions. Such movements are more likely to cause injury to your joints than more gentle movements.
- **Eat enough calories for the extra energy you need for both your pregnancy and exercise.** An additional 300 calories a day are usually required during pregnancy. You might need even more, depending on how much you exercise. Check with your medical caregiver to be sure.
- **Don't rotate your trunk while your hips or spine are flexed.** This can cause intervertebral disk injury.

In addition, you would be wise to

- rise slowly from the floor to avoid dizziness, and move around for a few moments after rising;
- begin slowly and advance gradually in your program if you've been sedentary;
- stop exercising and consult your medical caregiver if unusual symptoms appear (see "Warning Signs to Stop Exercising" on p. 35);
- not hold your breath while you exercise (many women tend to do this, especially during strenuous activity; this can reduce your oxygen supply and cause dizziness or fainting);
- return to your prepregnancy exercise routine slowly once you've given birth.

# EXERCISING SAFELY

We've talked about safe goals and guidelines in general. Now let's look at specifics: What conditions restrict exercise? What are warning signs to stop exercising? What activities are safe? Unsafe? What are guidelines for specific activities such as swimming, jogging, and strength training? How should you adapt your exercise through each trimester? In the next few pages we'll look at factors that affect your safety.

## CONDITIONS THAT RESTRICT EXERCISE

If you have any of the conditions listed below, you should not exercise vigorously—and it is possible that your medical caregiver may determine that any prenatal exercise is too risky for you. Stop exercising and contact your medical caregiver immediately if any of these conditions manifests itself during your pregnancy:

- Active myocardial disease (disease of the inner wall of the heart)
- Congestive heart failure
- Rheumatic heart disease
- Thrombophlebitus (vein inflamed with blood clot)
- Recent pulmonary embolism (blood clot in the lungs)

- Severe isoimmunization (for example, when an Rh-negative mother develops harmful antibodies to an Rh-positive baby's blood cells)
- Risk of premature labor
- Vaginal bleeding or ruptured membranes
- Intrauterine growth retardation
- Suspected fetal distress (as shown through a sonogram, reduced fetal movements, or fetal monitoring)

A note on fetal movement: Most women don't feel their baby moving until around weeks 18 to 21—and it may take longer before you can discern your baby's movement. When you are active, you tend to feel the movements less. Normally there is no need to count fetal movements, but your medical caregiver may have you do so if she or he feels you are at risk.

## WARNING SIGNS TO STOP EXERCISING

If you experience any of these signs, you should stop exercising immediately and contact your medical caregiver:

- Vaginal bleeding
- Abdominal or chest pain
- Leaking or gushing from vagina
- Sudden swelling of hands, face, or feet
- Severe, persistent headache
- Dizziness or lightheadedness
- Noticeable reduction in fetal activity
- Painful, reddened area in the leg
- Severe pain in pubic area or hips
- Pain or burning sensation when urinating
- Irritating vaginal discharge
- Oral temperature over 100 °F (38°C)
- Persistent nausea or vomiting
- Uterine contractions
- Heart palpitations
- Shortness of breath

## SAFE ACTIVITIES

The following activities are among the many that are safe; just keep in mind the ACOG guidelines and listen to your body. If you're too tired or nauseated, back off that day. If you feel you are overexerting, overheating, or becoming dehydrated, stop or slow down and make sure you get enough liquids. To monitor your exertion, use the talk test or the rate of perceived exertion (you shouldn't exceed the perception that you are exercising "somewhat hard") as well as pulse checks.

- **Walking**—Many call this the ideal exercise for pregnant women. Walking is recommended for women who have been sedentary.

- **Swimming**—Because it's a non-weight-bearing exercise and involves no ballistic movements or dangerous twists and turns,

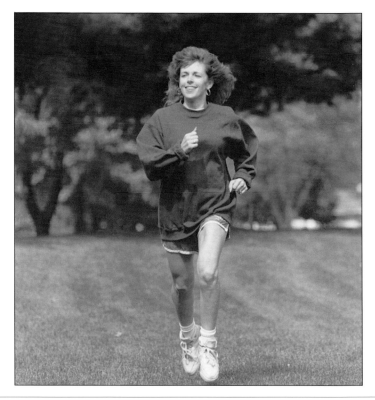

If you enjoyed jogging before your pregnancy, you can safely continue to improve your endurance by jogging throughout your pregnancy.

swimming is also ideal for pregnancy (although you shouldn't dive into the water). Swimming will help improve your endurance and tone your muscles.

- **Biking**—Biking is another good exercise for pregnant women because it is non-weight-bearing. Once your center of balance shifts, you should switch to a stationary bike.

- **Jogging**—While jogging is safe, most physicians recommend that you jog only if you have been jogging previously. Pay attention to signs of overheating and dehydration. Many women jog safely throughout their pregnancy.

- **Aerobic exercise classes**—High impact is out, but low impact is okay. It depends on the individual response; balance and strain on knees and back can be issues for some women, but in general, low-impact aerobics is safe.

- **Racquet sports**—If you're a tennis, badminton, or racquetball player, chances are you'll be fine playing your sport through your first two trimesters. In your third trimester, balance and lateral movement can become issues, and you may want to switch to walking, swimming, or some other activity.

- **Strength training**—Light weights are okay; heavy weights can cause problems with blood flow to the baby. If you don't overwork, however, weights can be a great way to strengthen muscles and joints, improve stability, and increase well-being.

You can also safely use rowing machines, stair climbers, and treadmills and partake in activities such as paddleball, Ping-Pong, and archery. Other activities that are generally safe but can cause balance problems—especially later in pregnancy—are softball, volleyball, cross-country skiing, step exercise, golf, and bowling.

If you're unsure about the safety of an activity, ask your medical caregiver.

## UNSAFE ACTIVITIES

These activities are deemed unsafe because they put you or your fetus at risk: skydiving, hang gliding, high diving, deep-sea diving, football, rugby, other contact sports, jumping feet first into water, downhill skiing, water skiing, surfing, horseback riding, field hockey, and basketball.

## GUIDELINES FOR SPECIFIC ACTIVITIES

Following are guidelines for four popular activities: walking and jogging (combined), swimming, and strength training.

### Walking and Jogging

- Wear good shoes that support your feet and cushion your legs from impact.
- Wear a good exercise bra and proper clothing. Remember that during your pregnancy you can overheat more quickly than before. In warm weather, wear cotton clothes that breathe.
- Warm up before you reach your target pace. If you're walking, walk more slowly to begin; if you're jogging, walk for a few minutes first.
- In warm climates, work out during the coolest part of the day.
- Drink plenty of water.
- Listen to your body. If you hurt, stop. If your perceived rate of exertion is high, slow down.
- Monitor your pulse and keep it in your target range.
- Avoid ice.
- Don't jog in sickness, pain, or in very hot or humid weather.

### Swimming

- Warm up by walking in the water or swimming slowly.
- Don't dive into the water.
- Slow your pace or shorten your workout if you feel fatigued.
- Monitor your pulse; keep it in your target heart range.
- Don't hold your breath while swimming.
- Listen to your body. If you hurt, stop.
- Try different strokes if you're uncomfortable. For example, try sidestroking if your back hurts.

- Don't jump in feet first; there's a small chance water may be forced into your vagina.
- Use flippers to help you kick. This is especially helpful late in your pregnancy.
- Don't swim alone.

## Strength Training

- If you haven't been weight training before, don't start during your pregnancy. Also, don't lift if you have problems with your muscles, joints, or bones, or if you have medical complications, such as high blood pressure or cardiovascular disease.
- Don't lift on consecutive days.
- Don't lift alone.
- Don't strain. Use light weights that you can lift 10 to 12 times fairly easily.
- Perform repetitions slowly, completing your full range of motion to increase flexibility. When you can perform 12 repetitions easily, add a little weight. Progress slowly.
- Don't hold your breath. Breathe slowly and evenly, exhaling as you lift, inhaling as you lower the weight.
- Stop when you feel your muscles "burn." Also, if an exercise is uncomfortable, don't do it.
- Lift using proper technique; don't sacrifice form to lift weights.
- Don't do hip or back exercises after the fourth month. If you have a bad back, don't do these exercises at all.
- Supplement your weight training with cardiovascular workouts, such as walking or swimming.

## Things to Avoid in Strength Training

- Wearing a tight belt around your belly.
- Lying flat on your belly.
- Performing hip abductor and adductor exercises after 16 weeks. (This will help you avoid arterial compression.)

- Doing leg extensions on any leg resistance machine. (This can be stressful if done improperly.)
- Performing leg curls, squats, or lunges.
- Using a duo hip and back machine or a 10-degree chest machine.
- Using a rotary torso or overhead press machine if you have back problems.

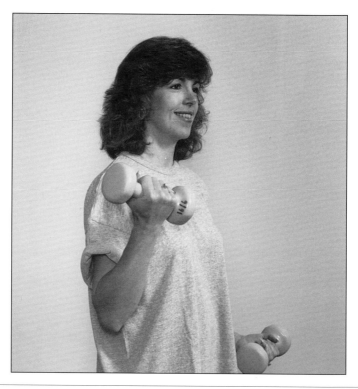

Never lift alone, and don't lift if you didn't before pregnancy. Use proper technique and light weights, and check other precautions with your medical caregiver.

## YOUR PRENATAL EXERCISE CHECKLIST

Before you begin your prenatal exercise program, read this common sense checklist—much of which is review of earlier material.

☐ Receive permission from your medical caregiver before taking part in a prenatal exercise class or working out on your own.

☐ If you're not already enrolled in prenatal exercise class, check with your local YMCA. The benefits of socialization and support, gained through working out with an instructor and with other pregnant women, can exceed the advantages of working out alone.

☐ Work out at least three times a week.

☐ Wear appropriate clothing; be especially careful in your first trimester not to overheat, which you will do more readily now that you're pregnant. Wear an exercise bra and supportive shoes.

☐ Always include warm-ups and cooldowns in your workouts.

☐ Following the exercise guidelines on pages 38-40; keep within your target heart range with a comfortable exertion level.

☐ Don't do exercises that cause you pain or discomfort.

☐ Check frequently for separation of your abdominal muscles (see the self-test on page 15) and do modified curl-ups if your muscles are separated by more than 1 in.

☐ Don't hold your breath when you exercise.

☐ Drink plenty of liquids and avoid exercising in hot, humid weather.

☐ Follow ACOG recommendations.

Remember, prenatal exercise should be safe and fun. It can benefit your health and fitness not only during your pregnancy but during your delivery and recovery. Work out wisely and enjoy the benefits!

# Part II

# EXERCISE PROGRAMS

n Part I you learned how exercising can help you during and after pregnancy, how the physiological changes of pregnancy affect exercise, and what types of activities are safe and unsafe. You also learned about the components that make up a sound exercise program and about setting healthy goals, including

- improving or maintaining cardiovascular fitness,
- maintaining muscle strength,
- improving flexibility,
- improving posture,

- improving general health, and
- having fun.

In Part II we present land and water programs to help you achieve those goals. Chapters 3 and 4 include a workout shell to be used as a guide in putting together your specific program; lists of stretching and strengthening exercises; and the exercises themselves, shown and described in detail. Chapter 5 shows you relaxation and breathing exercises that will help you during your pregnancy and especially during labor.

Remember to stretch and strengthen all major body areas in each workout. Your goal is to improve flexibility and maintain strength throughout your entire body. To help you do this, we've broken down the exercises by

- abdominals,
- arms/upper body,
- back,
- head/neck,
- legs/lower extremities, and
- pelvic floor.

Also note that, for comfort's sake, you should regularly alternate exercise positions—don't do more than a few exercises at a time in any one position (especially on your back). We recommend that you do your exercises in this progression: standing, sitting, on your back (if you're not past your third month), on your side, and on your hands and knees. It's not essential that you stick to this pattern, but do vary your position.

Be smart—listen to your body. You're not training for the Olympics; you're working out to maintain or improve your fitness and health, to help you feel good about and comfortable with your changing body, and to hasten your recovery from childbirth. Be consistent in your workouts, be safe, and have fun.

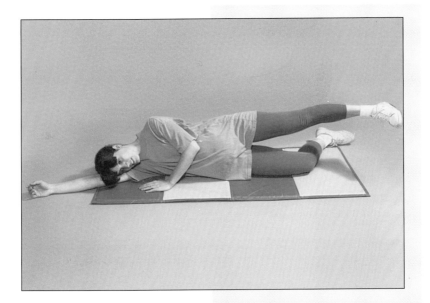

# Chapter 3

# Land Exercise

Use the following workout shell and list of exercises to shape a beneficial and safe program. Vary your exercises, working all major body areas, and alternate your positions within each workout. Remember that the American College of Obstetricians and Gynecologists recommends that you not do any exercises on your back after your first trimester of pregnancy.

Exercises done while lying on your back are denoted with an (*) to remind you to avoid such exercises after your first trimester. When an exercise can be done in more than one position, we list the alternative position in parentheses.

## INCORPORATING PELVIC FLOOR EXERCISES

The importance of doing pelvic floor exercises can't be overestimated. You can incorporate these exercises with other stretching and strengthening exercises; for example, as you're doing wall push-ups, you can also do a pelvic floor exercise, such as a contract and release or an elevator. Do at least three sets of pelvic floor exercises each workout, and try to do 50 repetitions each day.

| Component | Activity | Time |
|---|---|---|
| Warm-up | Walking or marching in place, pumping arms | 5 min |
| Aerobic | Walking or other aerobic activity chosen from pp. 36-37; use last 5 min as cooldown | 20 min |
| Strengthening | Four to six exercises from lists on pp. 47-48; incorporate a pelvic floor exercise | 10 min |
| Cooldown | Walking and slow, repetitive movements of major muscle groups; slacken pace; focus on deep breathing | 5 min |
| Stretching | Three to five stretches from lists on pp. 48-49; incorporate a pelvic floor exercise | 5 min |
| Relaxation | One exercise from chapter 5 | 5 min |

## STRENGTHENING EXERCISES

### ABDOMINALS

| Exercise | Position | Page |
|---|---|---|
| 1. Pelvic tilt | hands and knees (on back; on side) | 50 |
| 2. Hip hiking | on side | 51 |
| 3. Curl-up* | on back | 52 |
| 4. Modified curl-up* | on back | 53 |
| 5. Pelvic tilt with heel sliding* | on back | 54 |

### ARMS/UPPER BODY

| Exercise | Position | Page |
|---|---|---|
| 6. Biceps curl | standing (sitting) | 55 |
| 7. Triceps press | standing (sitting) | 56 |
| 8. Wall push-up | standing | 57 |
| 9. Butterfly press | standing (sitting) | 58 |

### BACK

| Exercise | Position | Page |
|---|---|---|
| 10. Arm raises | hands and knees | 59 |
| 11. Overhead pull-down | standing (sitting) | 60 |
| 12. Upright row | standing | 61 |
| 13. Bridging* | on back | 62 |

### HEAD/NECK

| Exercise | Position | Page |
|---|---|---|
| 14. Chin tucks | standing (sitting) | 62 |

## LEGS/LOWER EXTREMITIES

| Exercise | Position | Page |
|---|---|---|
| 15. Straight-leg raise | sitting | 63 |
| 16. Hip adduction | on side | 64 |
| 17. Hip abduction | on side | 65 |
| 18. Hip extension | hands and knees | 66 |

## PELVIC FLOOR

| Exercise | Position | Page |
|---|---|---|
| 19. Contract and release | any comfortable position | 67 |
| 20. Elevator | any comfortable position | 67 |
| 21. Super Kegels | any comfortable position | 67 |

# STRETCHING EXERCISES

## ARMS/UPPER BODY

| Exercise | Position | Page |
|---|---|---|
| 22. Shoulder circles | standing (sitting) | 68 |
| 23. Arm circles | standing (sitting) | 69 |
| 24. Upper chest stretch | sitting | 70 |
| 25. Triceps stretch | standing (sitting) | 71 |
| 26. Ladder climb | standing | 72 |

## BACK

| Exercise | Position | Page |
|---|---|---|
| 27. Cat back stretch | hands and knees | 73 |
| 28. Trunk turns | standing | 74 |
| 29. Lateral trunk stretch | standing | 75 |
| 30. Heel sits | hands and knees | 76 |
| 31. Hip rolls* | on back | 77 |
| 32. Baby-go-round | sitting | 78 |

## HEAD/NECK

| Exercise | Position | Page |
|---|---|---|
| 33. Neck bends | standing (sitting) | 79 |
| 34. Neck stretch | standing (sitting) | 80 |

## LEGS/LOWER EXTREMITIES

| Exercise | Position | Page |
|---|---|---|
| 35. Ankle circles | standing (sitting) | 81 |
| 36. Calf stretch | standing | 82 |
| 37. Buttocks stretch* | on back | 83 |
| 38. Hamstring stretch | sitting | 84 |
| 39. Inner thigh stretch | sitting | 85 |
| 40. Lunges | standing | 86 |
| 41. Leg swings | standing | 87 |
| 42. Straddle stretch | sitting | 87 |

## PELVIC FLOOR

| Exercise | Position | Page |
|---|---|---|
| 43. Pelvic floor relaxation* | on back | 88 |

# STRENGTHENING EXERCISES

| NO. 1  PELVIC TILT | ABDOMINALS |
|---|---|

**Purpose:** To strengthen your abdominal muscles, improve posture, and relieve strain on your back muscles.

**Starting position:** Standing with your back against a wall (if available), feet shoulder-width apart, and heels 12 to 18 in. from the wall with knees slightly bent.

**Movement:** Rotate your pelvis so your lower back comes in contact with the wall. Tighten your abdominal muscles and hold this "pelvic brace" position.

**Guidelines:** Hold 5 sec; repeat 10 times.

**Note:** Do not let your back sag forward when relaxing.

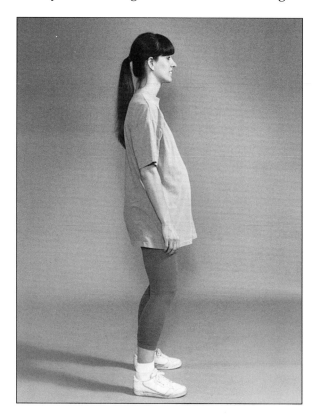

## NO. 2  HIP HIKING                    ABDOMINALS

**Purpose:**  To strengthen your lateral abdominal muscles.

**Starting position:**  Lying on your side with top leg straight, bottom leg bent, and head resting on outstretched bottom arm.

**Movement:**  Raise top leg 2 in. and hold in this position, then use lateral abdominal muscles to pull the hip toward the shoulder, keeping the top leg straight as you pull.

**Guidelines:**  Hold 5 sec; repeat 10 times; repeat with other leg.

**Note:**  When performing this exercise correctly, the top leg will move up toward the head while the bottom leg remains stationary.

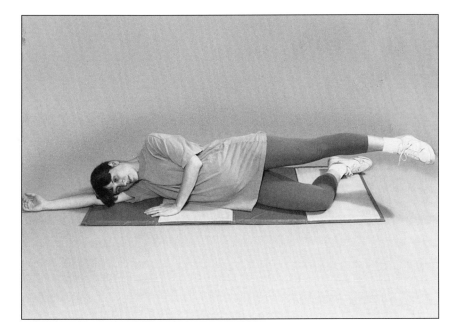

## NO. 3 CURL-UP*                               ABDOMINALS

**Purpose:** To strengthen your abdominal muscles.

**Starting position:** Lying on your back with knees bent.

**Movement:** Raise your head and shoulders and reach toward your knees with outstretched arms.

**Guidelines:** Repeat 10 times, three sets; progress by varying the arm positions:

- Arms across chest
- Hands touching sides of head, elbows out (do not close elbows in front of your face as you curl up, but instead lift your head and shoulders off the floor)

**Note:** Do not perform without checking for separation of your abdominal muscles first; perform only if they have not separated by more than 1 in. (see Self-Test for Abdominal Muscle Separation on p. 15).

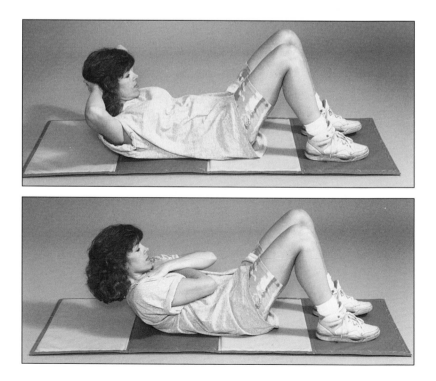

## NO. 4  MODIFIED CURL-UP*          ABDOMINALS

**Purpose:** To strengthen your abdominal muscles if they are separated by more than two fingers' width (see Self-Test for Abdominal Muscle Separation on p. 15).

**Starting position:** Lying on your back with knees bent and arms crossed over abdomen so that one wrist is above the other.

**Movement:** As you exhale, gently raise your head while keeping your shoulders on the floor; draw your arms together like a corset to support the abdominal muscles.

**Guidelines:** Repeat 10 times, three sets.

**Note:** Don't raise your shoulders because the separation in your abdominal muscles may increase.

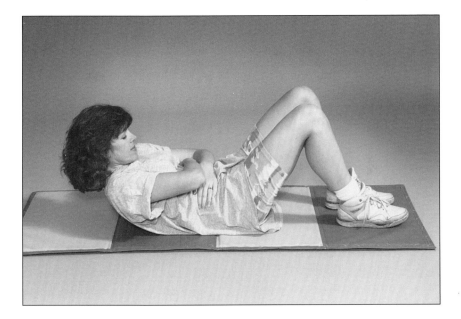

## NO. 5  PELVIC TILT WITH HEEL SLIDING*    ABDOMINALS

**Purpose:** To stabilize your back and strengthen your lower stomach muscles.

**Starting position:** Lying on your back with knees bent.

**Movement:** Perform a pelvic tilt, which will flatten your back, and hold it; slide one leg out as far as you can while maintaining the pelvic tilt.

**Guidelines:** Repeat 10 times with each leg; to progress, slide both legs out together, but return them one at a time.

**Note:** If you begin to lose the tilt, stop and return leg to starting position and relax tilt.

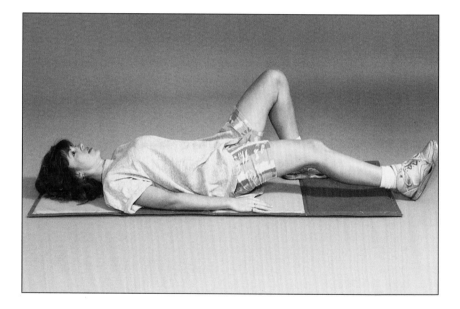

## NO. 6  BICEPS CURL | ARMS/UPPER BODY

**Purpose:** To strengthen the front muscles of your upper arms.

**Starting position:** Standing with arms at your sides, palms facing forward, knees relaxed.

**Movement:** Raise your hands toward your shoulders, bending at the elbow.

**Guidelines:** Repeat 10 to 15 times, three sets; progress by holding small weight (1 or 2 lb).

**Note:** As an alternative movement, raise your arms out to your sides at shoulder level, palms facing up, and bring hands toward the shoulders, bending arms at the elbows.

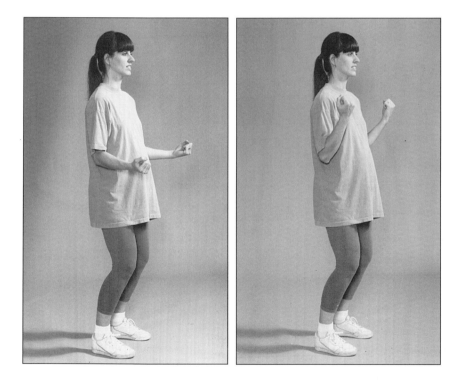

## NO. 7  TRICEPS PRESS                    ARMS/UPPER BODY

**Purpose:** To strengthen the back muscles of your upper arms.

**Starting position:** Standing with arms at sides, elbows bent, and knees slightly bent, bending forward slightly at the waist.

**Movement:** Push hands backward, extending the arms straight at the elbows.

**Guidelines:** Repeat 10 to 15 times, three sets; progress by holding small weights (1 or 2 lb).

**Note:** Keep elbows next to hips.

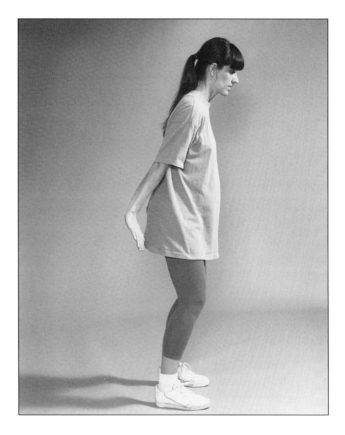

## NO. 8 WALL PUSH-UP ARMS/UPPER BODY

**Purpose:** To strengthen your upper arm and chest muscles.

**Starting position:** Standing facing the wall with hands flat on wall at shoulder level.

**Movement:** Slowly lower chest in toward the wall, bending your arms at the elbows; push back up by straightening arms. Keep feet flat on the floor and back and legs aligned throughout the movement.

**Guidelines:** Repeat 10 to 15 times; progress by standing farther from wall.

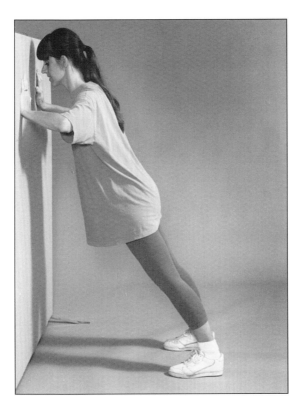

## NO. 9  BUTTERFLY PRESS                     ARMS/UPPER BODY

**Purpose:** To strengthen your upper chest muscles and stretch your shoulder blades.

**Starting position:** Standing, holding arms straight out to sides at shoulder level, elbows at 90-deg angle; keep knees slightly bent.

**Movement:** Pull arms together so forearms meet in front, resisting the movement by contracting your arm and chest muscles.

**Guidelines:** Repeat 10 to 15 times, three sets; progress by holding small weights (1 or 2 lb).

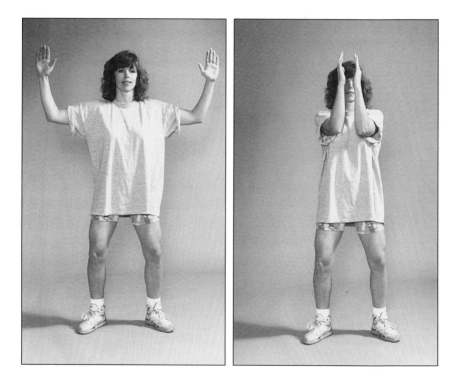

## NO. 10  ARM RAISES                                    BACK

**Purpose:** To strengthen your shoulder blade and upper back muscles.

**Starting position:** On hands and knees with back flat.

**Movement:** Raise one arm straight out in front to shoulder level and lower it.

**Guidelines:** Hold 5 sec; repeat 10 times with each arm; progress by placing 1- or 2-lb weights around wrists or holding weights.

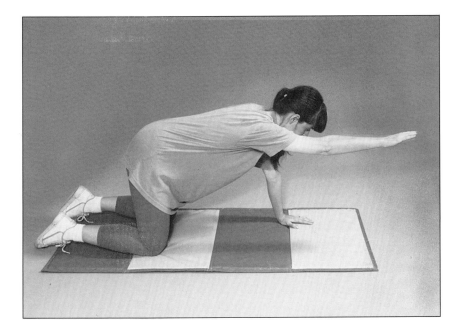

## NO. 11 OVERHEAD PULL-DOWN | BACK

**Purpose:** To strengthen your middle and lower back muscles.

**Starting position:** Standing with arms extended overhead; envision yourself holding onto a bar with both hands; keep knees relaxed.

**Movement:** Pull arms down together, bending elbows to the side until hands reach shoulder level, bringing the imaginary bar behind your head. Return arms to starting position.

**Guidelines:** Repeat 10 to 15 times, three sets; progress by holding 1- or 2-lb weights.

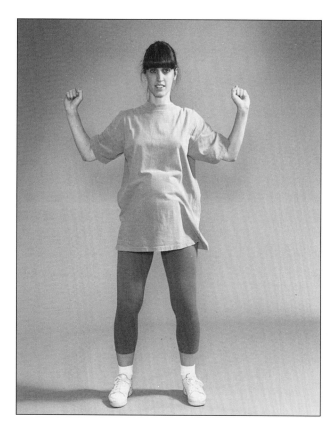

## NO. 12 UPRIGHT ROW | BACK

**Purpose:** To strengthen your lateral shoulder and upper back muscles.

**Starting position:** Standing with feet shoulder width apart and knees relaxed; arms at your sides with palms facing backward.

**Movement:** Pull elbows back and upward until they are at shoulder height, resisting the movement; then lower them to starting position (imagine you are holding a bar in front of your body as you lift).

**Guidelines:** Repeat 10 to 15 times, three sets; progress by holding 1- or 2-lb weights.

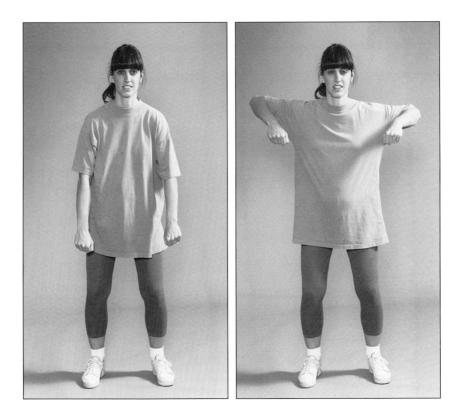

## NO. 13  BRIDGING*                                    BACK

**Purpose:** To strengthen your buttocks and to relieve pressure in the pelvic floor.

**Starting position:** Lying on your back with knees bent.

**Movement:** Perform a pelvic tilt (see exercise No. 1), lifting hips and buttocks off the floor until knees and chest form a straight line; keep the back straight.

**Guidelines:** Hold 5 sec; repeat 10 to 15 times; progress by moving feet farther away from buttocks (as you do so, squeeze harder with your buttocks so you rely less on your rear thigh muscles).

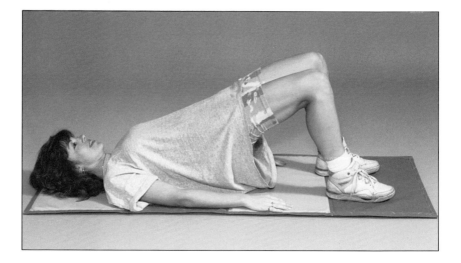

## NO. 14  CHIN TUCKS                                HEAD/NECK

**Purpose:** To strengthen your rear neck muscles and correct forward head posture.

**Starting position:** Standing or sitting in a comfortable position; keep knees relaxed.

**Movement:** Pull head straight back.

**Guidelines:** Hold 5 sec; repeat 5 times.

## NO. 15 STRAIGHT-LEG RAISE | LEGS/LOWER EXTREMITIES

**Purpose:** To strengthen your front thigh and hip muscles.

**Starting position:** In sitting position, leaning back on elbows with one leg bent and the other leg straight.

**Movement:** Slowly lift straight leg 8 to 10 in. off floor and slowly lower it.

**Guidelines:** Repeat 10 to 15 times, three sets, both legs; progress by adding 1- or 2-lb ankle weights.

**Note:** Women with back pain should sit up straight rather than lean on their elbows. Chin should be kept down.

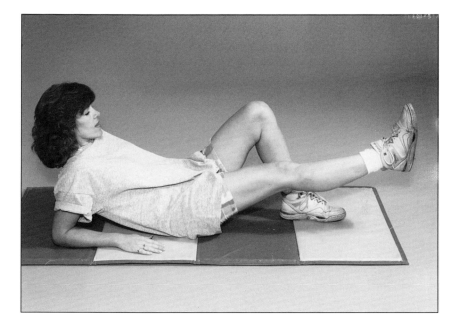

## NO. 16 HIP ADDUCTION — LEGS/LOWER EXTREMITIES

**Purpose:** To strengthen your inner thigh muscles.

**Starting position:** Lying on your side with top leg placed behind bottom leg with knees bent about 90 deg and foot flat on floor.

**Movement:** Slowly lift bottom leg 8 to 10 in. off floor and slowly lower it.

**Guidelines:** Repeat 10 to 15 times, three sets; repeat with other leg.

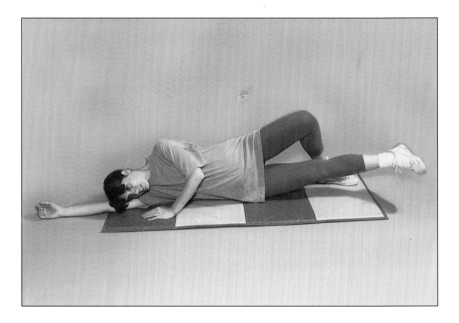

## NO. 17  HIP ABDUCTION   LEGS/LOWER EXTREMITIES

**Purpose:** To strengthen your outer thigh muscles.

**Starting position:** Lying on your side.

**Movement:** With bottom leg slightly bent and top leg straight, slowly lift top leg 8 to 10 in. and lower it.

**Guidelines:** Repeat 10 to 15 times, three sets; repeat with other leg.

**Note:** Alternative movements are:

- With hips and knees at 90-deg angle, lift top leg and lower it.
- With knees slightly bent, roll top knee toward ceiling and lower it.

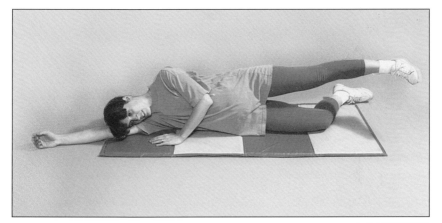

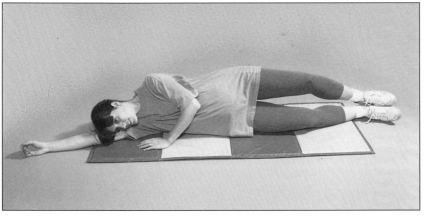

## NO. 18  HIP EXTENSION — LEGS/LOWER EXTREMITIES

**Purpose:** To strengthen your buttocks and rear thigh muscles.

**Starting position:** On hands (or forearms) and knees with back flat.

**Movement:** Straighten one leg behind you, keeping your knee straight and the supporting leg under the center of your body; slowly lift leg to buttock level and lower it.

**Guidelines:** Repeat 10 to 15 times, three sets; repeat with other leg.

**Note:** Don't allow your back to arch.

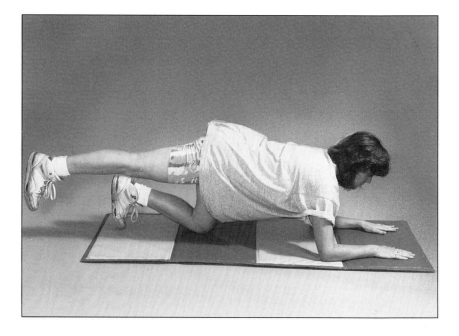

## NO. 19  CONTRACT AND RELEASE | PELVIC FLOOR

**Purpose:** To strengthen your pelvic floor muscles.

**Starting position:** Any comfortable position.

**Movement:** Draw up the pelvic floor, contracting the muscles, then releasing them.

**Guidelines:** Hold 3 to 5 sec; repeat 3 to 5 times frequently during the day.

**Remember:** The pelvic floor exercises should be done daily for the rest of your life; do only 3 to 5 at one time, but aim for 50 total each day.

## NO. 20  ELEVATOR | PELVIC FLOOR

**Purpose:** To strengthen your pelvic floor muscles.

**Starting position:** Any comfortable position.

**Movement:** Imagine you are in an elevator, and as you ascend to each floor, draw up the pelvic floor a little more; when you reach your limit, don't just let go, but instead gradually descend floor by floor.

**Guidelines:** Repeat 3 to 5 times frequently during the day.

**Remember:** The pelvic floor exercises should be done daily for the rest of your life; do only 3 to 5 at one time, but aim for 50 total each day.

## NO. 21  SUPER KEGELS | PELVIC FLOOR

**Purpose:** To strengthen your pelvic floor muscles.

**Starting position:** Any comfortable position.

**Movement:** Contract the pelvic floor muscles and hold them; renew the contraction if it fades.

**Guidelines:** Hold the contraction for 20 sec; repeat 1 to 2 times frequently during the day.

**Remember:** The pelvic floor exercises should be done daily for the rest of your life; do only 3 to 5 at one time, but aim for 50 total each day.

# STRETCHING EXERCISES

| NO. 22  SHOULDER CIRCLES | ARMS/UPPER BODY |
|---|---|

**Purpose:** To increase flexibility in your shoulders.

**Starting position:** Standing with arms at your sides and knees slightly bent.

**Movement:** Alternately circle shoulders back and down.

**Guidelines:** Repeat 10 times with each shoulder, slowly.

**Note:** Do not circle forward because this increases the tendency toward rounded shoulders.

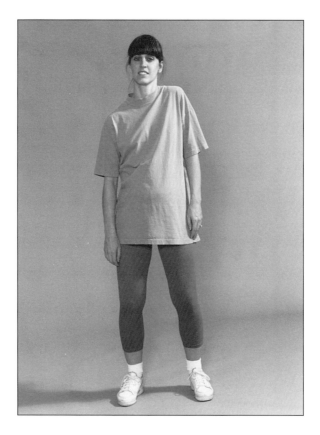

## NO. 23 ARM CIRCLES | ARMS/UPPER BODY

**Purpose:** To increase flexibility of the muscles in your rib cage, upper back, and shoulders.

**Starting position:** Standing with arms at your sides and knees slightly bent.

**Movement:** Circle both arms back; emphasize reaching up and back to open up the rib cage; keep elbows slightly bent while circling.

**Guidelines:** Repeat 10 times, slowly.

**Note:** Do not circle forward.

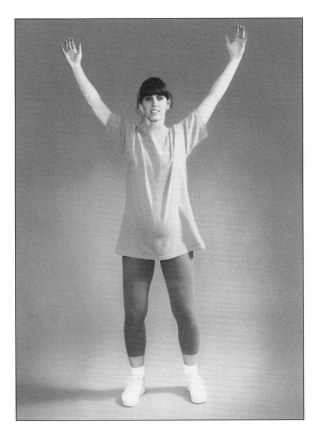

## NO. 24 UPPER CHEST STRETCH — ARMS/UPPER BODY

**Purpose:** To stretch your chest muscles and straighten rounded shoulders.

**Starting position:** Sitting in tailor position (spine erect with legs folded comfortably in front of your body) with hands clasped behind your back.

**Movement:** Lift arms up while squeezing shoulder blades together.

**Guidelines:** Hold 10 sec; repeat 10 times.

**Note:** Do not bend forward at the waist and do not bounce your arms.

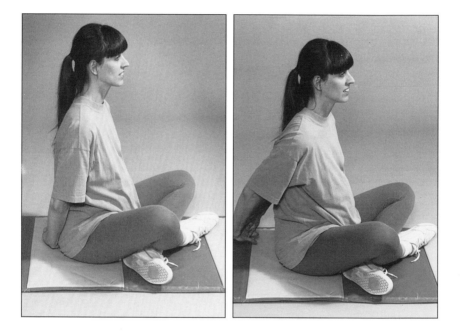

## NO. 25 TRICEPS STRETCH ARMS/UPPER BODY

**Purpose:** To stretch the rear muscles of your upper arms.

**Starting position:** Standing with arms at sides and knees relaxed.

**Movement:** Reach one hand overhead and toward the opposite shoulder blade.

**Guidelines:** Hold 10 to 15 sec; repeat 3 times with each arm.

**Note:** Do not bend at the waist and do not arch your back.

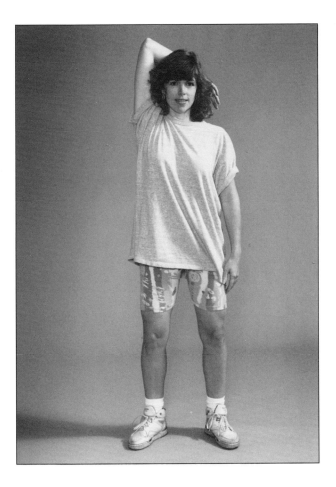

## NO. 26 LADDER CLIMB | ARMS/UPPER BODY

**Purpose:** To increase flexibility in your shoulders, arms, and lateral trunk muscles.

**Starting position:** Standing with arms overhead, knees and elbows slightly bent, or sitting.

**Movement:** Slowly reach up toward ceiling with first one hand and then the other; try to reach slightly higher with each repetition.

**Guidelines:** Repeat 10 times for each side.

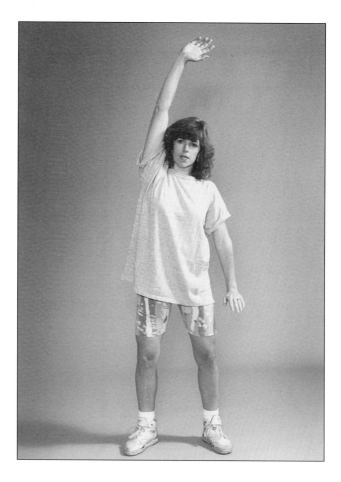

## NO. 27 CAT BACK STRETCH       BACK

**Purpose:** To stretch your entire back.

**Starting position:** On hands and knees with back flat.

**Movement:** Arch the back along the spine from tailbone up through shoulder blades; return to neutral position.

**Guidelines:** Hold 5 sec; repeat 5 times.

**Note:** Don't let your back sag when lowering. Hand position may cause discomfort for those with carpal tunnel syndrome; experiment by using knuckles or fingertips rather than palms.

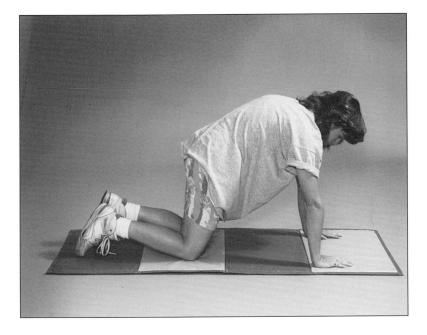

## NO. 28  TRUNK TURNS

**Purpose:** To increase flexibility in your trunk, hips, and shoulders.

**Starting position:** Standing with feet shoulder width apart and arms out to sides at shoulder level; keep knees and elbows slightly flexed.

**Movement:** Slowly swing your arms from side to side, allowing your head, shoulders, and trunk to follow; knees and feet should remain stationary.

**Guidelines:** Repeat 10 to 15 times in each direction.

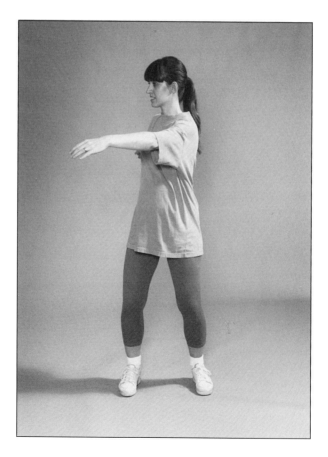

## NO. 29  LATERAL TRUNK STRETCH                      BACK

**Purpose:** To stretch your side trunk muscles, lateral hip muscles, and arms.

**Starting position:** Standing with feet shoulder width apart, one arm at your side and the other arm resting with hand on hip, knees slightly bent.

**Movement:** Lean toward the side with the hand on the hip and bring the opposite (free) arm overhead.

**Guidelines:** Hold 10 to 15 sec; repeat 3 to 5 times in each direction.

**Note:** Do not lean forward or backward during this stretch; later in your pregnancy, place your support hand lower on the hip.

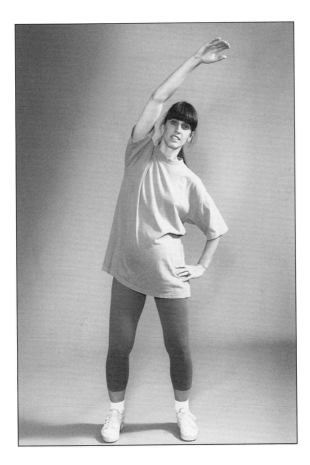

## NO. 30  HEEL SITS                                         BACK

**Purpose:** To stretch your lower back and buttocks.

**Starting position:** On hands and knees with knees spread wide.

**Movement:** Slowly rock back to sit on heels; as the baby grows, move knees wider apart to accommodate; while sitting back, walk fingers forward, increasing the stretch (stretch one arm at a time for greater flexibility).

**Guidelines:** Hold 20 to 30 sec; repeat 2 to 3 times.

**Note:** If you have knee problems, rock back only as far as comfortable for your knees. Raise up by sliding elbows toward knees and pushing up with legs.

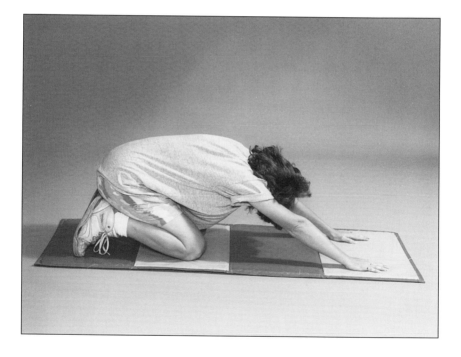

## NO. 31  HIP ROLLS*                          BACK

**Purpose:** To increase flexibility in your hips and stretch your back.

**Starting position:** Lying on your back with knees bent and arms stretched out at your sides.

**Movement:** Perform a pelvic tilt, flattening your back, then slowly move knees together toward floor; return to starting position and repeat on opposite side.

**Guidelines:** Hold 1 to 2 sec; repeat 10 times for each side.

**Note:** Arm position can be varied.

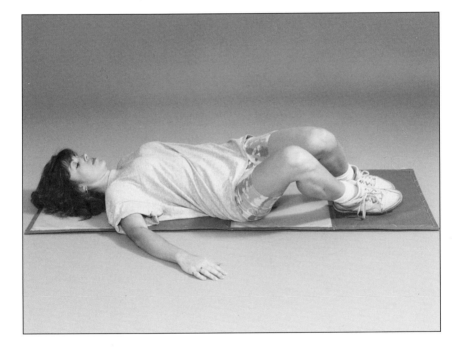

## NO. 32 BABY-GO-ROUND                    BACK

**Purpose:** To stretch your lower back.

**Starting position:** Tailor sitting with hands resting on knees or floor.

**Movement:** Bend forward, rounding the back, moving in one continuous circular motion.

**Guidelines:** Alternate directions; repeat 4 to 6 times.

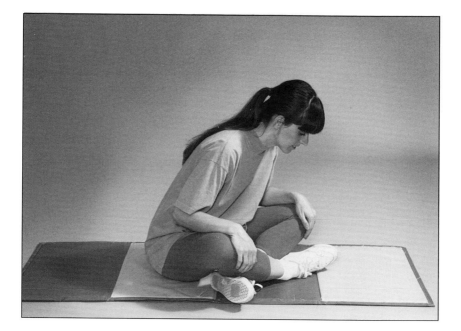

## NO. 33 NECK BENDS
HEAD/NECK

**Purpose:** To stretch your neck muscles.

**Starting position:** Standing or sitting in comfortable position (make sure knees are relaxed).

**Movement:** Drop chin to chest, feeling the stretch along the back of the neck, then lift head to upright position and drop ear to shoulder; repeat movement in opposite direction.

**Guidelines:** Hold each position 10 to 15 sec; repeat 5 times in each direction.

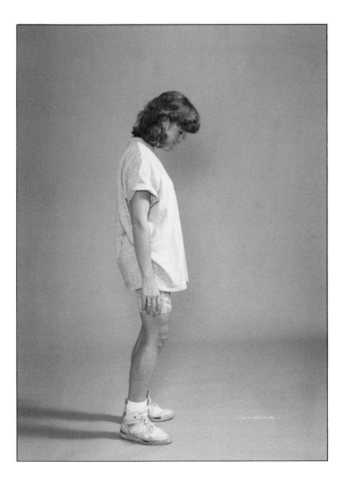

## NO. 34  NECK STRETCH
HEAD/NECK

**Purpose:** To stretch your neck muscles.

**Starting position:** Standing or sitting with one hand on opposite shoulder.

**Movement:** Slowly bend head sideways, away from the hand; press down on shoulder to increase the stretch.

**Guidelines:** Hold 15 sec; repeat 3 to 5 times for each side.

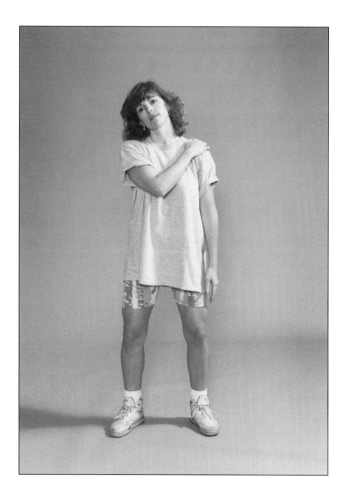

## NO. 35 ANKLE CIRCLES  |  LEGS/LOWER EXTREMITIES

**Purpose:** To loosen your ankles, improve circulation in your lower legs, and help prevent leg and foot cramps.

**Starting position:** Standing or sitting (keeping knees relaxed); if sitting, place leg on opposite knee.

**Movement:** Lift one foot off the floor and circle it clockwise and then counterclockwise; flex foot up and release.

**Guidelines:** Repeat 5 to 10 times in all directions with each foot.

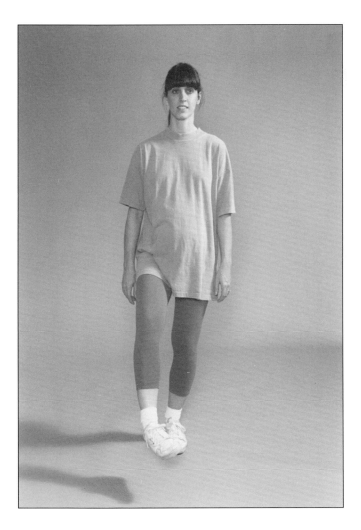

## NO. 36  CALF STRETCH          LEGS/LOWER EXTREMITIES

**Purpose:** To stretch the muscles in the back of the lower leg.

**Starting position:** Standing with hands on wall at shoulder level, one foot forward and one foot back.

**Movement:** Lean toward the wall, bending elbows slightly and keeping back leg straight with foot flat on the floor; keep both feet pointing toward wall.

**Guidelines:** Hold 20 to 30 sec; repeat 3 to 5 times with each leg; progress by increasing distance between your feet or leaning closer to the wall.

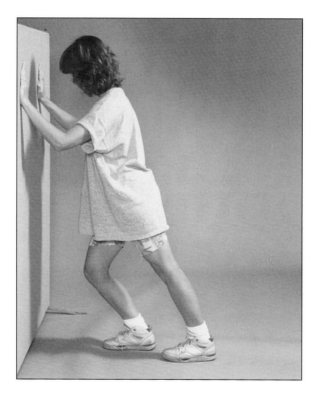

## NO. 37  BUTTOCKS STRETCH*    LEGS/LOWER EXTREMITIES

**Purpose:** To stretch your buttock and hip muscles.

**Starting position:** Lying on your back with knees bent and feet on
floor.

**Movement:** Place one foot on opposite knee and then bring that knee
toward your chest; tighten abdominal muscles as you lift the leg.

**Guidelines:** Hold 10 to 15 sec; repeat 3 to 5 times with each leg; as
pregnancy progresses and it becomes difficult to bring knee toward chest, you can slide the foot closer to the buttock to achieve
the stretch.

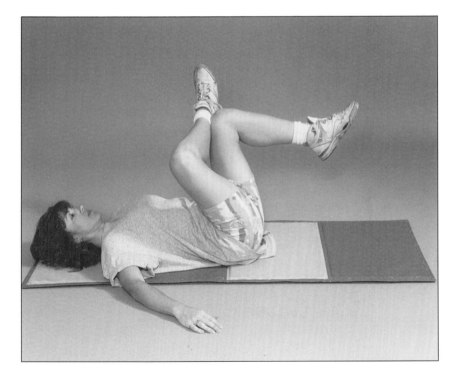

## NO. 38 HAMSTRING STRETCH    LEGS/LOWER EXTREMITIES

**Purpose:** To stretch your rear thigh muscles.

**Starting position:** Sitting with one leg straight and the other leg bent with heel in toward the straight leg, hands placed behind buttocks for support.

**Movement:** Stretch your spine upward and then lean forward toward straight leg.

**Guidelines:** Hold 20 to 30 sec; repeat 3 to 5 times with each leg.

**Note:** Do not let shoulders round forward; bend from the hips, not the waist.

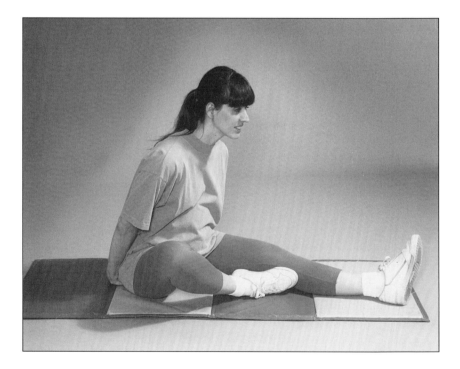

## NO. 39  INNER THIGH STRETCH   LEGS/LOWER EXTREMITIES

**Purpose:** To stretch your inner thigh muscles.

**Starting position:** Sitting up straight with soles of feet together, hands behind buttocks for support.

**Movement:** Stretch your spine upward and allow your knees to relax toward the floor; focus on lengthening your spine from the pelvis to the neck.

**Guidelines:** Hold 20 to 30 sec; repeat 3 to 5 times.

**Note:** Don't pull feet in toward your body, and don't do this stretch if you have pubic pain because it may aggravate it.

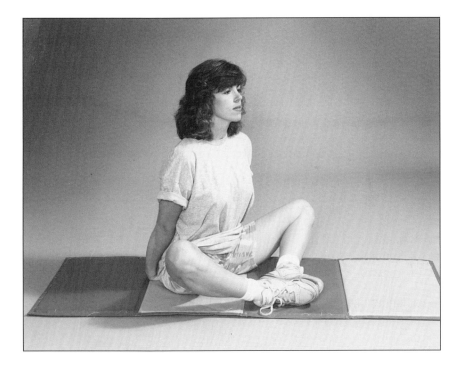

## NO. 40  LUNGES

**LEGS/LOWER EXTREMITIES**

**Purpose:** To stretch your inner thigh and pelvis.

**Starting position:** Standing with legs greater than shoulder width apart and hands resting on thighs.

**Movement:** Slowly lunge toward one side, then return to starting position and move in the opposite direction.

**Guidelines:** Hold 5 sec; repeat 5 to 10 times in each direction.

**Note:** Keep knees over feet.

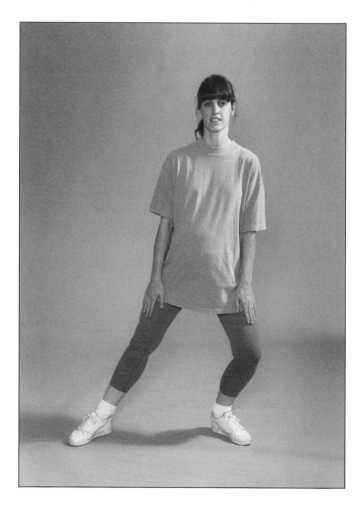

## NO. 41  LEG SWINGS | LEGS/LOWER EXTREMITIES

**Purpose:** To stretch your hip muscles and improve balance and coordination.

**Starting position:** Standing on one leg with arm on that side holding onto the wall for balance.

**Movement:** Swing the free leg front to back and then side to side in a controlled yet relaxed manner.

**Guidelines:** Do 10 times each direction with each leg.

**Note:** Do not allow foot of supporting leg to roll inward; keep supporting leg slightly bent.

## NO. 42  STRADDLE STRETCH | LEGS/LOWER EXTREMITIES

**Purpose:** To stretch your inner thigh muscles.

**Starting position:** Sitting with legs spread apart as far as comfortable, hands behind buttocks for support.

**Movement:** Stretch tall by lengthening the spine and roll feet outward, feeling the stretch in your inner thigh.

**Guidelines:** Hold 20 to 30 sec; repeat 3 to 5 times.

## NO. 43 PELVIC FLOOR RELAXATION*            PELVIC FLOOR

**Purpose:** To relax your pelvic floor muscles.

**Starting position:** Lying on your back with knees bent and soles of feet together (pillows can be placed under knees for support).

**Movement:** Slowly relax knees toward floor, opening up the pelvic floor and inner thighs; slowly contract the pelvic floor muscles for 3 sec, hold for 3 sec, then relax for 3 sec; hold the relaxation for 30 to 60 sec and then bring knees back up.

**Guidelines:** Repeat 3 to 5 times.

**Note:** If position with knees apart is uncomfortable for lower back, perform a pelvic tilt (see exercise No. 1).

**Remember:** The pelvic floor exercises should be done daily for the rest of your life; do only 3 to 5 at one time, but aim for 50 total each day.

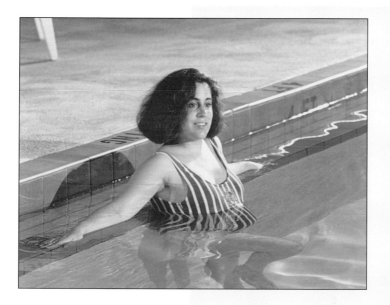

# Chapter 4

# Water Exercise

I f you're like most pregnant women, you'll find that exercising in water can be both comfortable and enjoyable. Many women who feel awkward on land feel quite adept in the water. The bouyancy feels good, and pain associated with weight-bearing activities is diminished.

A few notes before you begin your aquatic exercise:

- Stand in chest-deep water unless otherwise noted.

- Stand in shoulder-deep water for upper body exercises; keep your arms under water for arm exercises.

- Use slower movements for the stretching exercises, faster movements for the strengthening exercises.

- Use the edge of the pool or the ladder as needed for support.

- For side-to-side movement, stand with feet shoulder width apart and flat on the floor; for front-to-rear movement, stand with one leg in front of your body and one leg behind.

- Keep your knees slightly flexed for all exercises, and flex your wrists when using equipment.

- Cup your palms for arm exercises (to increase the resistance).

- Realize that when you exercise your arms and legs, you are using your back muscles and abdominals to stabilize yourself—this will tone those muscles as well.

- Useful equipment includes aqua joggers, paddles, barbells, cuff weights, water wings, and kickboards (depending on what equipment you have available, you may have to alter some exercises).

---

### INCORPORATING PELVIC FLOOR EXERCISES

The importance of doing pelvic floor exercises can't be overemphasized. You can incorporate these exercises with other stretching and strengthening exercises; for example, as you're doing wall push-ups, you can also do a pelvic floor exercise, such as a contract and release or an elevator. Do at least three sets of pelvic floor exercises each workout, and try to do 50 repetitions each day.

---

Use the following workout shell and list of exercises to shape a beneficial and safe program. Remember to vary your exercises and work all major body areas.

| Component | Activity | Time |
|---|---|---|
| Warm-up | Walking in pool, pumping arms | 5 min |
| Aerobic | Deep water jogging, swimming, or jogging in shallow water; use last 5 min as cooldown | 20 min |
| Strengthening | Four to six exercises from lists on pp. 91-93; incorporate a pelvic floor exercise | 10 min |
| Cooldown | Walking and slow, repetitive movements of major muscle groups; slacken pace, focus on deep breathing | 5 min |
| Stretching | Three to five stretches from lists on pp. 93-94; incorporate a pelvic floor exercise | 5 min |
| Relaxation | One exercise from chapter 5 | 5 min |

## STRENGTHENING EXERCISES

### ABDOMINALS

| Exercise | Page |
|---|---|
| 1. Pelvic tilt | 95 |
| 2. Side bends | 96 |
| 3. Reverse curl-up | 97 |

## ARMS/UPPER BODY

## BACK

## HEAD/NECK

## LEGS/LOWER EXTREMITIES

## PELVIC FLOOR

# STRETCHING EXERCISES

## ARMS/UPPER BODY

## BACK

## HEAD/NECK

## LEGS/LOWER EXTREMITIES

# STRENGTHENING EXERCISES

| NO. 1 PELVIC TILT | ABDOMINALS |
|---|---|

**Purpose:** To strengthen your stomach muscles, improve posture, and relieve strain on back muscles.

**Starting position:** Either standing against wall or free-standing.

**Movement:** Tuck under your buttocks and tilt your pelvis back, decreasing the curve in your lower back.

**Guidelines:** Hold 5 sec; repeat 10 times.

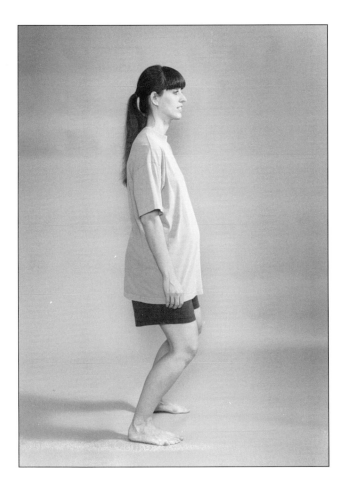

## NO. 2  SIDE BENDS                     ABDOMINALS

**Purpose:** To strengthen your side stomach muscles and lower torso.

**Starting position:** Standing in chest-deep water with arms at sides, holding paddles (optional).

**Movement:** Keeping arms straight, bend as far as possible to one side and return; repeat in other direction.

**Guidelines:** Repeat 10 to 15 times each direction.

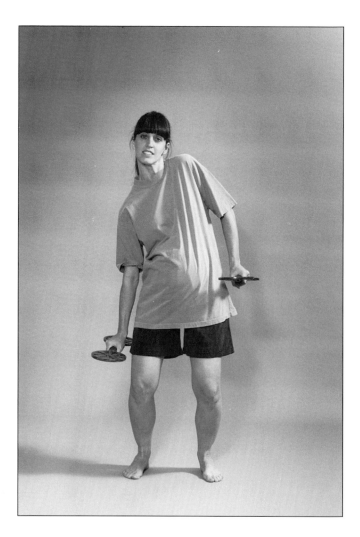

## NO. 3  REVERSE CURL-UP                    ABDOMINALS

**Purpose:** To strengthen your stomach muscles.

**Starting position:** Floating on your stomach, grasping pool edge with one hand, and placing the other hand lower on the pool wall; lift feet off floor and let them float behind you.

**Movement:** Perform a pelvic tilt and hold; pull knees toward your chest and then straighten them out.

**Guidelines:** Repeat 10 to 15 times, 3 sets.

**Note:** Leg movements can be performed separately.

## NO. 4  BICEPS CURL                    ARMS/UPPER BODY

**Purpose:** To strengthen the front muscles of your upper arms.

**Starting position:** Standing in chest-deep water with arms at your sides.

**Movement:** Raise hands toward shoulders by bending the elbows, palms open and facing upward.

**Guidelines:** Repeat 10 to 15 times, 3 sets.

**Note:** Progress by holding onto paddles.

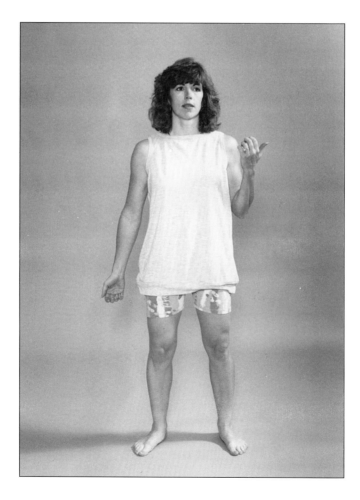

## NO. 5 ARM PRESS　　　　　ARMS/UPPER BODY

**Purpose:** To strengthen your upper chest muscles.

**Starting position:** Standing in neck-deep water with arms out to the sides and palms facing forward.

**Movement:** Press arms together in front of your body, palms touching each other.

**Guidelines:** Repeat 10 to 15 times, 3 sets.

**Note:** Increase the resistance by tensing the arm and chest muscles or by holding paddles.

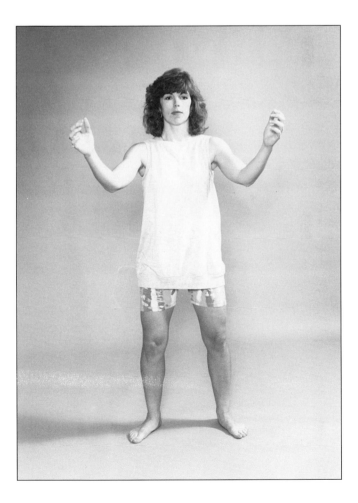

## NO. 6 TRICEPS PRESS                    ARMS/UPPER BODY

**Purpose:** To strengthen the rear muscles of your upper arms.

**Starting position:** Standing in chest-deep water with arms in front of your body, one hand on top of the other, elbows bent and pointing out to the sides.

**Movement:** Press hands down, with movement taking place at the elbows.

**Guidelines:** Repeat 10 to 15 times, 3 sets.

**Note:** Progress by holding paddles.

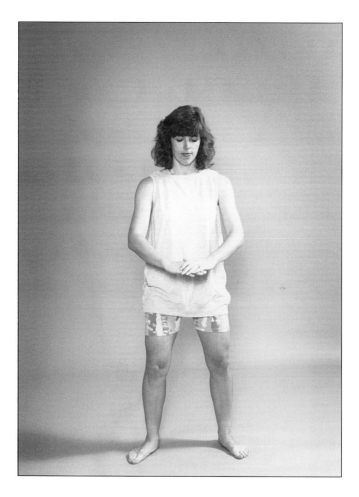

## NO. 7 LATERAL SHOULDER RAISES ARMS/UPPER BODY

**Purpose:** To strengthen the middle shoulder muscles.

**Starting position:** Standing in chest-deep water with arms at your sides.

**Movement:** Keeping arms straight, raise them out to your sides to just below the water's surface, palms down.

**Guidelines:** Repeat 10 to 15 times, 3 sets.

**Note:** Progress by holding paddles.

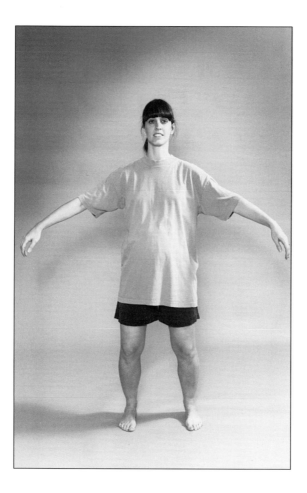

## NO. 8 ARM RAISES                              ARMS/UPPER BODY

**Purpose:** To strengthen the muscles in the front and back of your shoulders.

**Starting position:** Standing in chest-deep water with arms at your sides.

**Movement:** Keeping arms straight, raise them forward to just below the water's surface, palms up; then lower and raise them backward, palms down.

**Guidelines:** Repeat 10 to 15 times, 3 sets.

**Note:** Progress by holding paddles.

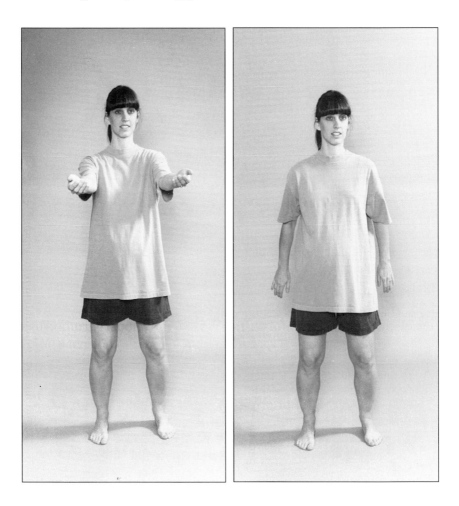

## NO. 9  PULL-DOWNS                                     BACK

**Purpose:** To strengthen your shoulder and upper back muscles.

**Starting position:** Standing in chest-deep water with arms to the front of your body and elbows slightly bent.

**Movement:** Keeping arms straight, pull down toward hips, palms down.

**Guidelines:** Repeat 10 to 15 times, 3 sets.

**Note:** Progress by holding paddles.

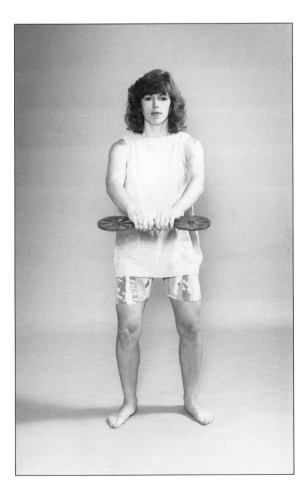

## NO. 10  BENT-OVER ROWING  `BACK`

**Purpose:** To strengthen your shoulder blade muscles and lower back.

**Starting position:** Standing in chest-deep water with body bent forward at the waist and arms slightly in front of you.

**Movement:** Pull arms backward, raising elbows toward ceiling.

**Guidelines:** Repeat 10 to 15 times, 3 sets.

**Note:** Progress by holding paddles.

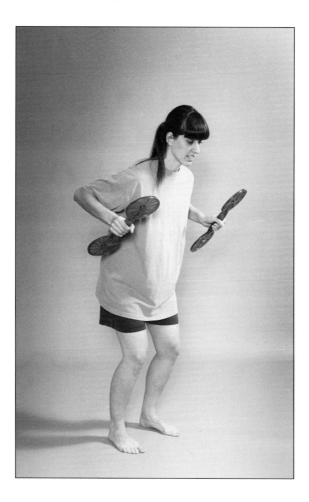

## NO. 11  STRAIGHT–LEG DEEP KICK BACK

**Purpose:** To strengthen your lower back and hip muscles.

**Starting position:** Standing in chest-deep water with back against pool wall, holding onto edge with arms straight out to sides.

**Movement:** Keeping back straight, alternately raise and lower legs.

**Guidelines:** Repeat 10 to 15 times, 3 sets.

**Note:** Progress by adding ankle weights.

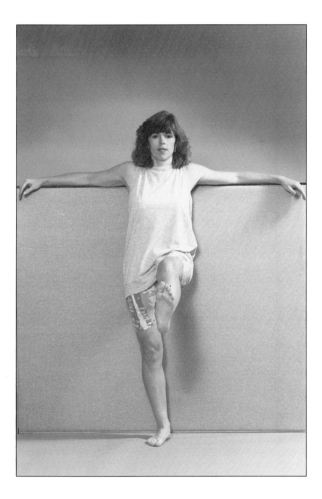

## NO. 12  TRUNK ROTATION WITH BAR                    BACK

**Purpose:** To strengthen your back and trunk muscles.

**Starting position:** Standing in chest-deep water holding onto bar in front of body.

**Movement:** Keeping back and trunk stabilized, twist body side to side as one unit.

**Guidelines:** Repeat 10 to 15 times, 3 sets.

**Note:** Paddles may be used in place of bar.

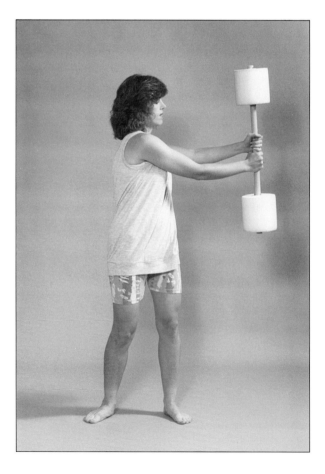

## NO. 13  CHIN TUCKS    HEAD/NECK

**Purpose:** To strengthen your rear neck muscles and correct forward head posture.

**Starting position:** Standing in comfortable position.

**Movement:** Pull head straight back.

**Guidelines:** Hold 5 sec; repeat 5 times.

## NO. 14 SHOULDER SHRUGS                    HEAD/NECK

**Purpose:** To strengthen upper shoulder muscles.

**Starting position:** Standing in chest-deep water with arms at your sides.

**Movement:** Shrug shoulders up and then push down.

**Guidelines:** Repeat 10 to 15 times, 3 sets.

**Note:** Progress by holding paddles.

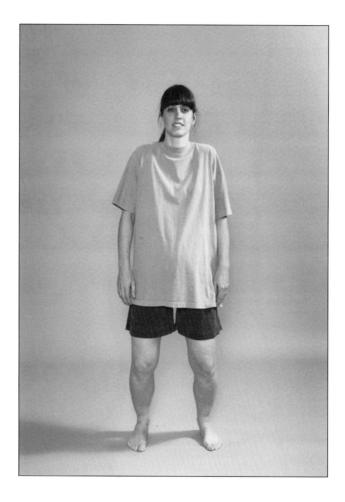

## NO. 15  HIP ROTATIONS  LEGS/LOWER EXTREMITIES

**Purpose:** To strengthen your hip rotator muscles.

**Starting position:** Standing with left side to pool wall and right foot on left leg, just above or below the knee, holding onto pool edge for support.

**Movement:** Swing right knee out and then in; turn to other side and repeat with opposite leg.

**Guidelines:** Repeat 10 to 15 times, 3 sets.

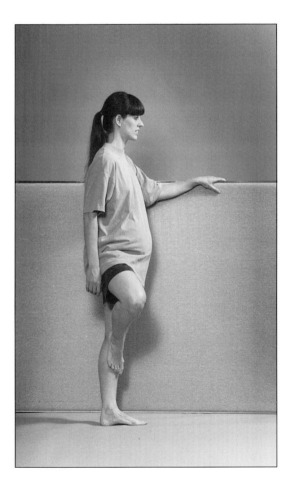

## NO. 16 HIP SWINGS            LEGS/LOWER EXTREMITIES

**Purpose:** To strengthen your side hip and inner thigh muscles.

**Starting position:** Standing in waist-deep water, sideways to pool wall and holding on for support.

**Movement:** Swing right leg out (about 2 ft, or to a comfortable distance) to the side and then pull it back in; repeat with opposite leg.

**Guidelines:** Repeat 10 to 15 times, 3 sets.

**Note:** Progress by moving away from pool wall or by adding ankle weights.

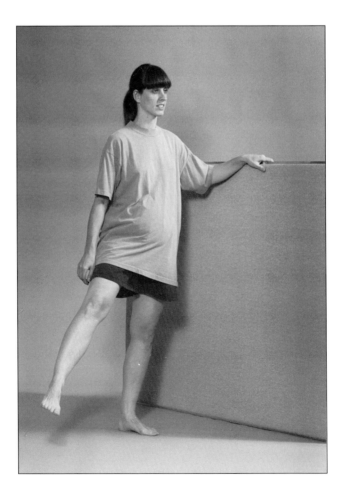

## NO. 17  BICYCLE

**LEGS/LOWER EXTREMITIES**

**Purpose:** To strengthen your hips, buttocks, and thighs.

**Starting position:** Floating on back with floats on arms.

**Movement:** Alternately bend and straighten your legs as if pedaling a bicycle.

**Guidelines:** Repeat 20 to 30 sec, 3 to 5 sets.

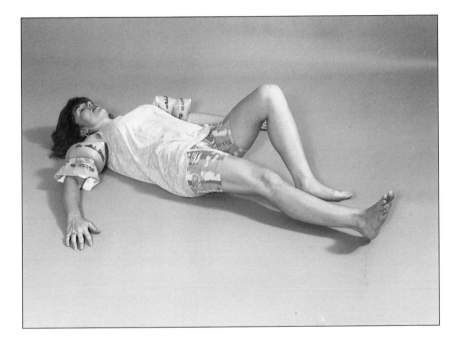

## NO. 18 STRAIGHT-LEG WALKING   LEGS/LOWER EXTREMITIES

**Purpose:** To strengthen front thigh muscles.

**Starting position:** Standing in waist-deep water.

**Movement:** Walk with little or no knee flexion.

**Guidelines:** Walk back and forth two pool lengths.

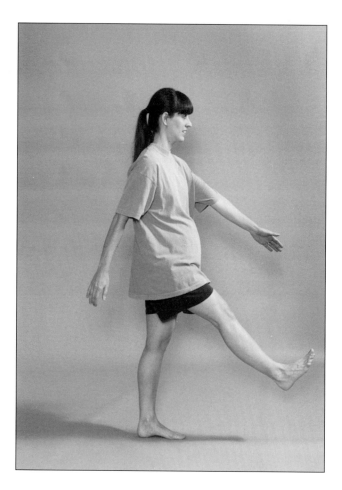

## NO. 19  CONTRACT AND RELEASE PELVIC FLOOR

**Purpose:** To strengthen your pelvic floor muscles.

**Starting position:** Any comfortable position.

**Movement:** Draw up the pelvic floor, contracting the muscles, then releasing them.

**Guidelines:** Hold 3 to 5 sec; repeat 3 to 5 times frequently during the class or out of the pool.

## NO. 20  ELEVATOR PELVIC FLOOR

**Purpose:** To strengthen your pelvic floor muscles.

**Starting position:** Any comfortable position.

**Movement:** Imagine you are in an elevator, and as you ascend to each floor, draw up the pelvic floor a little more; when you reach your limit, don't just let go, but instead gradually descend floor by floor.

**Guidelines:** Repeat 3 to 5 times frequently during the class or out of the water.

## NO. 21  SUPER KEGELS PELVIC FLOOR

**Purpose:** To strengthen your pelvic floor muscles.

**Starting position:** Any comfortable position.

**Movement:** Contract the pelvic floor muscles and hold them; renew the contraction if it fades.

**Guidelines:** Hold the contraction for 20 sec; repeat 1 to 2 times frequently during the class or out of the pool.

# STRETCHING EXERCISES

| NO. 22  LADDER CLIMB | ARMS/UPPER BODY |

**Purpose:** To stretch your side and shoulder muscles.

**Starting position:** Standing with arms at your sides.

**Movement:** Reach toward ceiling, one arm at a time.

**Guidelines:** Hold 3 to 5 sec; repeat 10 times each side.

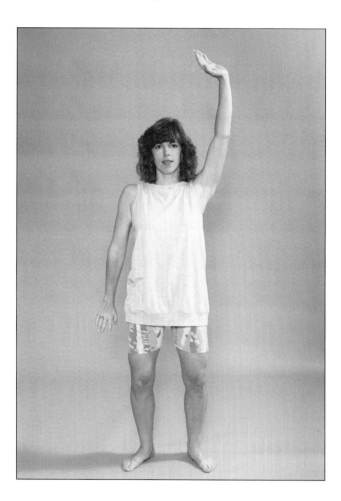

## NO. 23 SHOULDER CIRCLES | ARMS/UPPER BODY

**Purpose:** To stretch your shoulders.

**Starting position:** Standing with arms relaxed at your sides.

**Movement:** Alternately circle shoulders back and down.

**Guidelines:** Repeat 10 times each shoulder, slowly.

**Note:** Do not circle forward because this increases the tendency toward rounded shoulders.

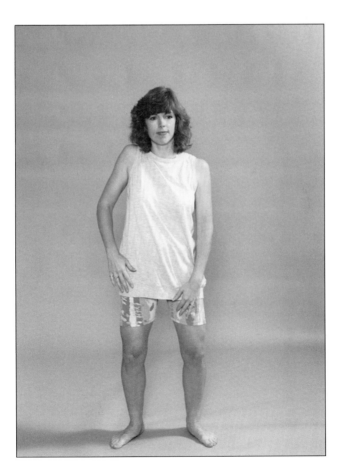

## NO. 24　HUGGIES　　　　　　　ARMS/UPPER BODY

**Purpose:** To stretch your upper back and shoulders.

**Starting position:** Standing with arms relaxed at your sides.

**Movement:** Stretch arms across your body, hugging yourself; bend knees as you hug; straighten legs as you release hug.

**Guidelines:** Hold 10 to 15 sec; repeat 5 times.

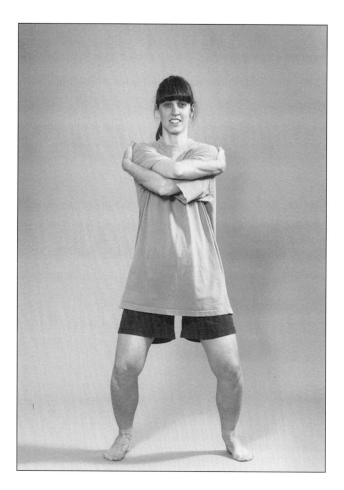

## NO. 25  ELBOW PRESS                     ARMS/UPPER BODY

**Purpose:** To stretch your upper back and chest.

**Starting position:** Standing with hands clasped behind head and elbows out to the sides.

**Movement:** Pull elbows back and then bring them together in front.

**Guidelines:** Hold each position 5 to 10 sec; repeat 5 times.

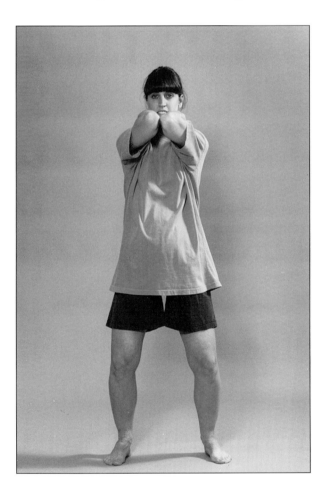

## NO. 26  WAITER'S BOW                                      BACK

**Purpose:** To stretch your upper and lower back.

**Starting position:** Standing facing the wall with hands holding onto edge of pool and arms fully extended.

**Movement:** Bend forward at the hips, keeping your back flat; go as far as comfortable, keeping your head above water.

**Guidelines:** Hold 5 to 10 sec; repeat 3 to 5 times.

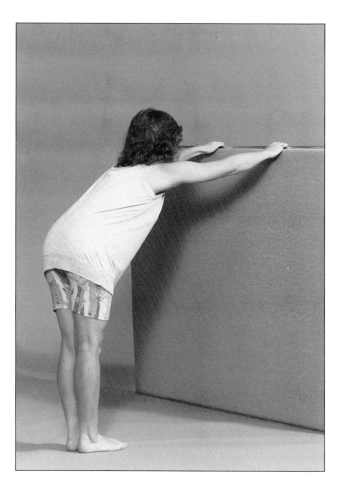

## NO. 27  LATERAL TRUNK STRETCH                    BACK

**Purpose:** To stretch your side trunk, lateral hip, and arm muscles.

**Starting position:** Standing with feet shoulder width apart and arms at your sides.

**Movement:** Bend to the right, bringing left arm overhead; bend to the left, bringing right arm overhead.

**Guidelines:** Hold each position 10 to 15 sec; repeat 3 to 5 times each direction.

**Note:** Do not lean forward.

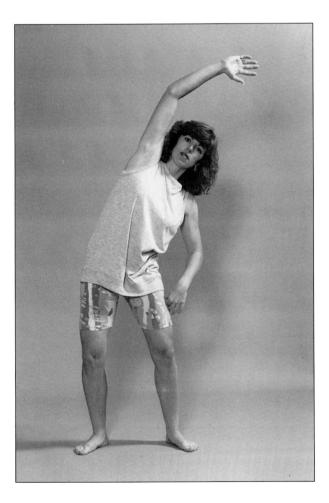

## NO. 28  TRUNK TURNS                                    BACK

**Purpose:** To stretch your trunk, hips, and shoulders.

**Starting position:** Standing with feet shoulder width apart and arms straight out to sides at shoulder level.

**Movement:** Slowly swing arms from side to side, allowing your head, shoulders, and trunk to follow.

**Guidelines:** Repeat 10 to 15 times each direction.

**Note:** Keep knees and feet stationary and pointing forward.

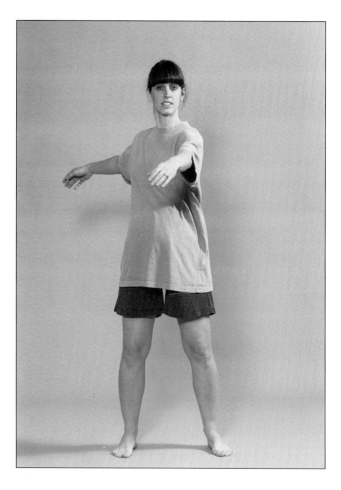

## NO. 29  HIP AND BACK STRETCH

**Purpose:** To stretch your hip extensors and lower back.

**Starting position:** Standing in chest-deep water with floats on your arms (or placing back against pool wall and reaching over your shoulders to grasp pool edge).

**Movement:** Bend your knees, one at a time, lifting them toward your chest.

**Guidelines:** Hold 5 to 10 sec; repeat 10 times.

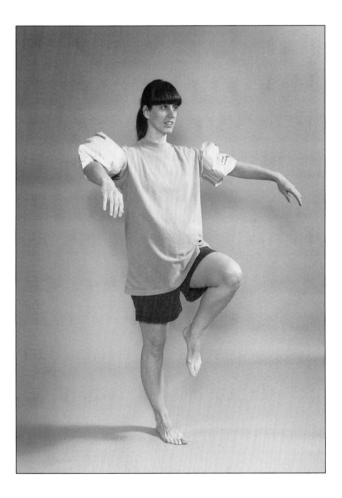

## NO. 30  NECK BENDS

HEAD/NECK

**Purpose:** To stretch your neck muscles.

**Starting position:** Standing in a comfortable position.

**Movement:** Drop chin to chest, feeling the stretch along the back of the neck, then lift head to upright position and drop ear to shoulder; repeat this movement in opposite direction.

**Guidelines:** Hold each position 10 to 15 sec; repeat 5 times each direction.

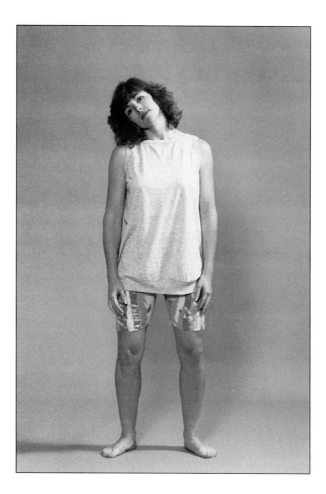

## NO. 31  NECK STRETCH                    HEAD/NECK

**Purpose:** To stretch your neck muscles and relieve tension in the neck.

**Starting position:** Standing with one hand placed on opposite shoulder.

**Movement:** Slowly bend head sideways, away from the hand; press down on shoulder to increase the stretch.

**Guidelines:** Hold 10 to 15 sec; repeat 3 to 5 times each side.

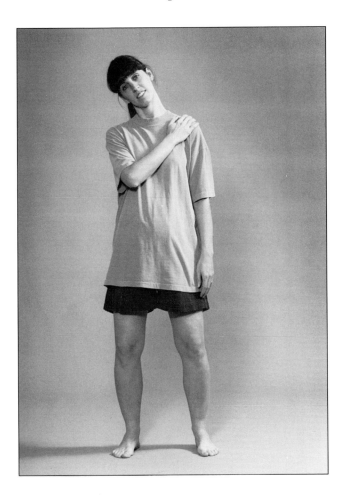

| NO. 32 ANKLE CIRCLES | LEGS/LOWER EXTREMITIES |
|---|---|

**Purpose:** To loosen your ankle joints and improve circulation in your lower legs.

**Starting position:** Standing.

**Movement:** Lift one foot and circle it clockwise and then counter-clockwise; flex foot up and relax it.

**Guidelines:** Repeat 5 to 10 times in all directions with each foot.

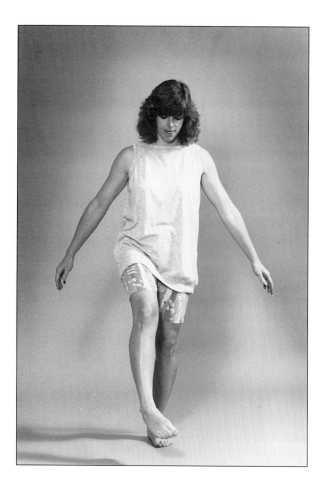

## NO. 33  CALF STRETCH | LEGS/LOWER EXTREMITIES

**Purpose:** To stretch your calf muscles.

**Starting position:** Standing facing pool wall, hands on wall for support.

**Movement:** Take small steps away from wall, going back as far as possible, keeping heels on floor; lean hips forward for added stretch.

**Guidelines:** Hold 20 to 30 sec; repeat 3 to 5 times for each leg.

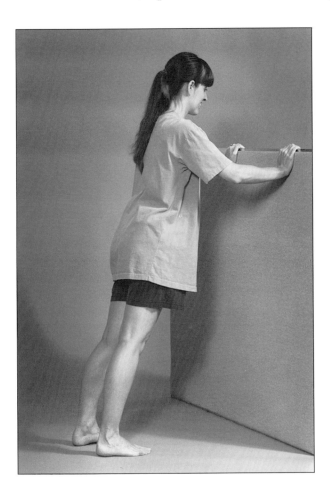

## NO. 34 AQUA LUNGE
### LEGS/LOWER EXTREMITIES

**Purpose:** To stretch your inner thighs.

**Starting position:** Facing pool wall and holding onto edge with both hands shoulder width apart; place feet in straddle position on the wall.

**Movement:** Slowly shift weight to one side, bending that knee; repeat in opposite direction.

**Guidelines:** Hold 10 to 15 sec; repeat 3 to 5 times for each leg.

**Note:** Keep feet flat on the wall.

## NO. 35  HAMSTRING STRETCH  | LEGS/LOWER EXTREMITIES

**Purpose:** To stretch your hamstring muscles.

**Starting position:** Standing on one leg with the other foot on ladder, wall, or step, keeping your knee straight.

**Movement:** Bending from waist, reach toward your toes.

**Guidelines:** Hold 20 to 30 sec; repeat 3 to 5 times for each leg.

**Note:** If you're unable to keep your knee straight, lower your foot slightly.

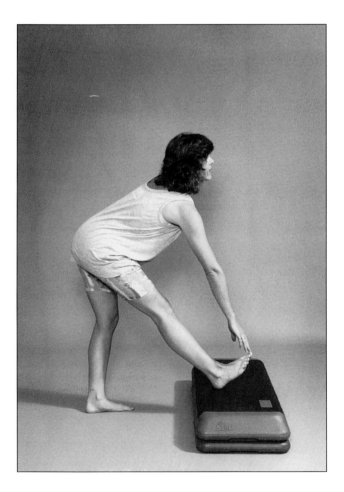

## NO. 36 QUADRICEPS STRETCH | LEGS/LOWER EXTREMITIES

**Purpose:** To stretch your front thigh (quadriceps) muscles.

**Starting position:** Standing with one side toward pool wall, holding onto wall for support; with the other hand, hold opposite ankle behind body.

**Movement:** Pull ankle toward buttocks while keeping hips pressed forward.

**Guidelines:** Hold 20 to 30 sec; repeat 3 to 5 times for each leg.

**Note:** Do not bend forward or rotate hips.

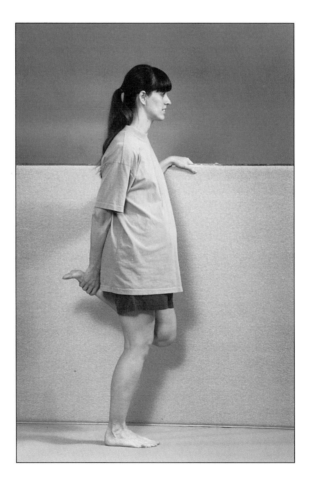

## NO. 37 LEG SWIRL                     LEGS/LOWER EXTREMITIES

**Purpose:** To stretch your hip muscles.

**Starting position:** Standing with one side toward pool wall, holding onto pool edge with one hand.

**Movement:** Slowly do circles with the outside leg, keeping it straight with the foot relaxed.

**Guidelines:** Repeat 5 to 10 times, both clockwise and counterclockwise, with both legs.

**Note:** Swing your leg from your hip; keep your upper body motionless.

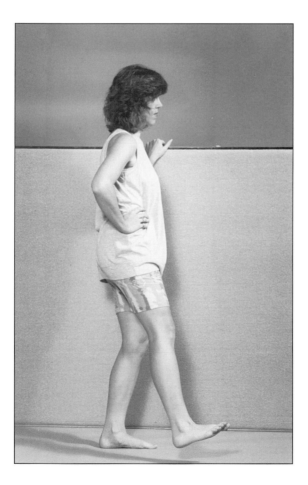

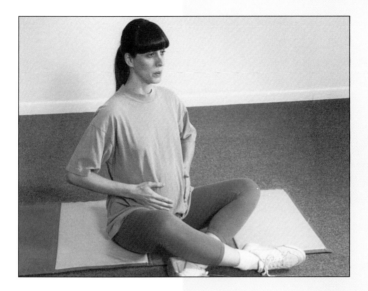

# Chapter 5

# Relaxation and Breathing Exercises

Relaxation techniques and breathing exercises are vital components of a prenatal exercise program. The exercises in this
chapter can help you release muscular and mental tension,
lessen fatigue and conserve energy, and reduce stress and calm your
mind.

More important, they can help you be in control of your pain
during childbirth and labor:

- By using proper breathing techniques, you ensure that your
  uterus—which is contracting during labor—gets adequate oxygen. When a muscle is oxygen-deprived, it hurts more.

- By employing relaxation skills, you can decrease tension and fatigue, which intensify pain.
- By focusing on relaxing and breathing properly, your attention is off your pain.

On the next few pages, we'll describe three effective ways to relax: through progressive relaxation, massage, and visualization. These exercises are best done when your muscles are slightly fatigued; do them at the end of your workout.

Before doing any of the exercises, get in a comfortable position—perhaps lying on your side, supported by a cushion or pillow, or sitting—and make sure your joints are slightly flexed and supported.

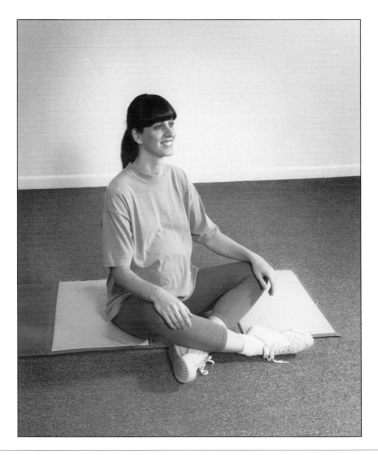

Relaxation exercises can reduce stress and calm your mind. They are best done at the end of your workout, when muscles are slightly fatigued.

# RELAXATION EXERCISE

## PROGRESSIVE RELAXATION

**Objective.** To slowly relax all the muscles in your body.

**Instruction.** Have your partner or a friend read this exercise to you in a slow, even voice. You should breathe slowly and evenly throughout, and close your eyes if it helps you concentrate.

---

Take a deep cleansing breath; breathe in through your nose, bringing the air into your lungs, down into your abdomen; now bring it up, exhaling through your mouth.

Take another cleansing breath.

As you exhale, feel your tension float away with your breath. Feel yourself growing calm.

We're going to concentrate on different muscles today, first tensing them and then releasing the tension. You want your limbs to become loose and floppy, to be totally relaxed.

We'll start at the top and move downward. When I mention a muscle or an area, you'll tense it and hold the tension for 10 sec. Then you'll release that tension and let it float away.

Tighten your forehead. Scrunch the muscles together by frowning hard. (*Wait 10 sec.*) Now release that tension.

Clench your jaw. Feel how tense it is. (*Wait 10 sec.*) Now release that tension. (If you have a temporomandibular disorder —TMD—skip this part.)

Stiffen your shoulders by moving them upward. Hold that tension . . . now release it. Feel how relaxed your shoulders are.

■

Clench your right arm and make a fist. Feel how the muscles in the forearm are tightened . . . now release it. Feel the muscles soften.

■

Now clench your left arm and make a fist . . . and release it.

■

Tighten your abdomen . . . and release it.

■

Tighten your hips and your bottom . . . and release the tension.

■

Now contract your pelvic floor . . . and release.

■

Stiffen the muscles in your right leg and foot by pointing your toes toward your body . . . and release.

■

Stiffen the muscles in your left leg and foot; point your toes toward your body . . . and release.

■

Check your whole body to make sure no tension has returned. Stay relaxed and take several cleansing breaths.

■

Okay, we're finished. Open your eyes and then rise slowly; otherwise you might feel dizzy or lightheaded.

---

Variation.  Touch relaxation is a valuable variation of progressive relaxation. You tense and release the same muscles in the same order as in progressive relaxation, but no verbal cues are given. Instead, you begin by tensing your forehead; your partner, seeing that tension, places his or her hand on your forehead and leaves it there until feeling the tension melt away.

The touch should be gentle but firm. This exercise is useful because, during labor, your partner can use touch relaxation to help you release tension.

# RELAXATION EXERCISE

## MASSAGE

**Objective.** To release tension and soothe aching muscles.

**Instruction.** Get in a comfortable position with your joints slightly flexed and supported; it may help to have a pillow under your head and neck, one between your knees, and one supporting your belly if you are lying on your side.

Your partner should try different types of massage:

- Stroking—Either light or firm strokes on tense areas, moving from the center of your body outward. On more tender areas, use lighter strokes. If any type of touch causes you discomfort or pain, your partner should stop that movement. Massage shouldn't hurt.

- Rubbing and kneading—Squeezing and releasing, done to the neck, shoulders, back, thighs, feet, and hands. Your partner

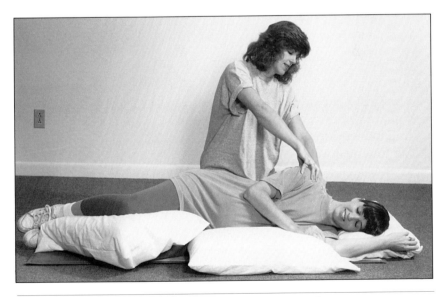

Massage can release tension and soothe aching muscles.

should use his or her thumbs to knead fleshy areas such as the buttocks. Again, your partner should be directed by what feels good to you.

- Effleurage—Light, feathery touching or stroking. If this is ticklish or uncomfortable for you, the strokes can be more firm. This technique is especially relaxing done in a circular motion over the lower abdomen.

Your partner might start with light strokes and progress to deeper strokes and kneading, as comfort dictates. Good places to massage include the feet (which often get tired during pregnancy), the back, the shoulders, and the head (many expectant mothers suffer from sinus headaches).

Varicose veins shouldn't be massaged; they should be stroked very lightly, and the strokes should be toward the heart. And your partner should use only flat, gentle strokes on your abdomen.

# RELAXATION EXERCISE 3

## VISUALIZATION

Objective.   To relax by picturing a pleasant scene. Our example is a walk on the beach, but you can use any scene that is relaxing to you.

Instruction.   This exercise can be combined with a body relaxation, as follows, or you can do a "body check" to make sure your muscles are relaxed before you begin your visualization. You can either do the exercise by yourself or have your partner read it to you. Closing your eyes may help you visualize the scene better. Either way, go slowly.

---

Relax by taking several cleansing breaths; breathe in through your nose, bringing the air deep into your lungs, into your abdomen, and now bring it up and exhale through your mouth.

Feel the tension melt away as you exhale.

■

Take another cleansing breath. Feel yourself grow calm as you exhale.

■

Concentrate on your facial muscles, your jaw, and your forehead. Release any tension you have there. Feel these muscles soften.

■

Release the tension in your neck and shoulders. As the tension melts away, feel the warmth that enters into your neck and shoulders.

■

Now feel that warmth as it travels down your arms and into your hands, which are completely limp. All tension is released from your hands and arms.

■

Now concentrate on your upper back. Relax your back.

■

Now relax your lower back. Feel how the muscles are warm, soft, and loose.

■

Now feel this warmth and softness in your abdomen. Totally relax your abdomen.

■

Let any tension drift away from your hips and your bottom.

■

Now relax your vaginal muscles. Feel them soften and grow warm.

■

Release any tension in your legs and feet. They should feel deliciously heavy and warm.

■

Take a cleansing breath. Check your body to make sure all your muscles are relaxed.

■

Take another cleansing breath. Breathe in through the nose, into the lungs and abdomen, exhale through the mouth. All tension in your body has drifted away. Now we're going to visualize.

■

You are walking along a seashore. For the moment you are on dry sand. You feel the warm grains of sand on the soles of your feet and between your toes. The warmth feels good.

■

A slight breeze blows through your hair. It's a warm breeze. You can smell the sea: fish and kelp, salt and sand. The breeze also brings the scent of pine from the trees just beyond a dune.

■

The sky is blue and streaked with white clouds. You look out on the water and see rolling waves, endlessly rolling.

■

You hear a seagull cry overhead. Several gulls walk along ahead of you on the sand. A few flap their wings a time or two as they walk, but they don't take off.

■

You walk closer to the water. You reach the wet sand, and it feels good and cool on your feet.

■

A wave rolls over your feet, washing salt water over them. You reach down and pick up a seashell and put it to your ear. You hear a distant roar that mimics the sea.

■

The sun warms your bare shoulders, washing over them in waves of heat. The warmth of the sun on your shoulders and the coolness of the water on your feet are soothing.

■

You carry the shell with you as you continue your walk. Up ahead, you hear the shouts of children. They are building sand castles.

■

As you near the gulls, they take a few quick steps, flap their wings, and fly away.

■

The motion of the gulls causes one of the children, a small girl, to look your way. Spotting you, she smiles and waves. You smile and wave back.

■

You feel peaceful and restful. The sun warms your face and makes you drowsy, yet you feel energetic, strong, alive.

■

The child runs up to you and you give her the seashell. She smiles in gratitude, looks at it, and puts it to her ear.

■

As you continue walking, she walks with you.

■

*(Pause longer than normal here.)*

■

Now close the exercise with a few cleansing breaths. Keep your body relaxed, and open your eyes. Remember to get up slowly.

The following exercises will help you control your pain during labor and delivery. They will help you relax, increase your concentration, and help ensure that all your muscles are receiving the oxygen they need. During labor, you can use these breathing exercises along with the relaxation skills you've just learned. You'll be able to concentrate better if you use an internal or external focal point as you breathe.

Begin and end all breathing exercises with a cleansing breath, which is the first exercise described. The exercises described here are not designed to be used during any specific part of labor; vary your patterns as needed to enhance your relaxation and concentration.

# BREATHING EXERCISE

# 1

## CLEANSING BREATH

The cleansing breath should be used to begin and end each breathing exercise—and each contraction during labor.

Take in a long, slow breath through your nose; feel it fill your chest and go down into your lower abdomen. Pause for a second or two and then exhale through your mouth. (If you are congested, do all the breathing through your mouth.)

## BREATHING EXERCISE

### SLOW CHEST BREATHING

This breathing is slow and rhythmic, done with a relaxed, slightly open mouth. Begin with a cleansing breath—breathe in deeply through your nose and exhale through your mouth.

Then breathe in evenly and fully through your nose, although not as deeply as for the cleansing breath. As you inhale, count from one to five, then exhale through your mouth, counting back down from five to one. Take eight of these breaths per minute.

## BREATHING EXERCISE

### MODIFIED SLOW CHEST BREATHING

Modified slow chest breathing is done at twice the rate of slow chest breathing: 16 breaths/min. This is approximately the rate of normal breathing.

## BREATHING EXERCISE

### PATTERN-PACED BREATHING

Pattern-paced breathing is done at the same rate as modified slow chest breathing—16 breaths/min—but it employs a rhythmic pattern of blowing out at regular intervals. The rhythmic blowing can have a calming effect and enhance your concentration. Try a 3:1 pattern (in-out, in-out, in-out, in-BLOW) or a 4:1 pattern (adding one more in-out before the blow). You might also try repeating words in rhythm to the pattern, such as "I-will, be-calm," or "Health-y, ba-by."

## BREATHING EXERCISE

### SHALLOW CHEST BREATHING

Shallow chest breathing is not as deep as slow chest breathing; it is a more rapid, rhythmic breathing. It may be hard to do at first; your mouth may get dry and you may feel out of breath, but keep practicing because it will be helpful during your labor.

Breathe in through your mouth, bringing the air about halfway down your chest, and exhale through your mouth. Take 1 breath/sec for 1 min; do this exercise 5 times a day.

If you breathe in too deeply, you might hyperventilate (exhale too much carbon dioxide). While this isn't serious, it will leave you feeling lightheaded and dizzy. If you feel these symptoms, cup your hands in front of your nose and mouth and breathe deeply for a few minutes.

## BREATHING EXERCISE

### MODIFIED SLOW/SHALLOW BREATHING

Modified slow/shallow breathing combines modified slow chest and shallow chest breathing. This can help you during the middle stage of labor while not exhausting you during the beginning or end stages. Begin (as always) with a cleansing breath, then do modified slow chest breathing at a rate of 16 breaths/min. After 15 sec of this, switch to shallow chest breathing—1 breath/sec—for 30 sec. Then return to modified slow chest breathing for 15 sec before finishing with a cleansing breath.

## BREATHING EXERCISE

### MODIFIED SHALLOW BREATHING

This exercise is especially helpful as your contractions get stronger. Take a cleansing breath and then begin shallow chest breathing (60 breaths/min). Pick up speed, working up to 120 breaths/min. Then slow back down to 60 breaths/min and close with a cleansing breath.

## BREATHING EXERCISE

### SHALLOW BLOW BREATHING

Shallow blow breathing consists of four shallow breaths followed by a blow: in-out, in-out, in-out, in-BLOW. Speed up or slow down the pace as necessary; as your contractions intensify you'll want to go faster.

## BREATHING EXERCISE

### ADVANCED SHALLOW BLOW BREATHING

This is similar to shallow blow breathing, but it involves varying patterns that help you concentrate and take your mind off the pain. After a cleansing breath, begin with three shallow breaths and a blow, as described in the previous exercise. Then try two shallow breaths and a blow, one and a blow, and move back up to three and a blow. Try the variations in this time frame: First 15 sec, 3:1; Next 15 sec, 2:1; Next 15 sec, 1:1; Next 15 sec, 2:1; Next 15 sec, 3:1.

# Bibliography

American College of Obstetricians and Gynecologists. (1985). *Exercise during pregnancy and the postnatal period.* Washington, DC: Author.

American College of Obstetricians and Gynecologists. (1990). *ACOG guide to planning for pregnancy, birth, and beyond.* Washington, DC: Author.

American College of Obstetricians and Gynecologists. (1992, October). Women and exercise. *ACOG Technical Bulletin #173.*

American College of Obstetricians and Gynecologists. (1994, February). Exercise during pregnancy and the postpartum period. *ACOG Technical Bulletin #189.*

Appel, C. (1992). Feeling fit. *Lamaze 1992 Parents' Magazine,* pp. 32-35.

Artal, R., Friedman, M., & McNitt-Gray, J. (1990, September). Orthopedic problems in pregnancy. *The Physician and Sportsmedicine,* pp. 93-105.

Artal-Mittelmark, R., Wiswell, R., & Drinkwater, B. (1991). *Exercise in pregnancy.* Baltimore: Williams & Wilkins.

Bing, E. (1992). Is it safe to have sex during pregnancy? *Lamaze 1992 Parents' Magazine,* pp. 21-23.

Brodey, D. (1993, November). Building bigger babies. *American Health,* p. 88.

Clapp, J. (1990). Exercise in pregnancy: A brief clinical review. *Fetal Medicine Review,* **2,** 89-101.

Cooper, M., & Cooper, K. (1972). *Aerobics for women.* New York: J.B. Lippincott.

Gaines, M. (1993). *Fantastic water workouts.* Champaign, IL: Human Kinetics.

Gauthier, M. (1986, April). Guidelines for exercise during pregnancy: Too little or too much? *The Physician and Sportsmedicine,* pp. 162-169.

Goliszek, A. (1987). *Breaking the stress habit.* Winston-Salem, NC: Carolina Press.

Graham, J. (1991). *Your pregnancy companion.* New York: Pocket Books.

Hage, M. (1992). *The back pain book*. Atlanta: Peachtree.

Holstein, B. (1988). *Shaping up for a healthy pregnancy: Instructor guide*. Champaign, IL: Human Kinetics.

*Human Nutrition Information Service* (1992). The food guide pyramid. United States Department of Agriculture HG Bulletin 252.

Hunt, J. (1993, September/October). Pregnant pause: Should expectant mothers hold off on exercise? *American Fitness*, pp. 44-45.

Infante-Rivard, C., Fernandez, A., Guthier, R., David, M., & Rivard, G.-E. (1993). Fetal loss associated with caffeine intake before and during pregnancy. *Journal of the American Medical Association*, **270**(24), 2940-2943.

Jiminez, S. (1992). Growing pains. *Childbirth Annual Magazine*, pp. 32-33.

Johnson, C. (1989). *Backstrokes*. Havertown, PA: Occupational Therapy Associates.

Katz, J. (1995). *The pregnant woman's complete guide to water fitness*. Champaign, IL: Human Kinetics.

Keith, C., & Sperling, D. (1984). *The birthing book*. New York: Times Books.

Kitzinger, S. (1989). *The complete book of pregnancy*. New York: Alfred A. Knopf.

Melpomene Institute. (1990). *The bodywise woman*. New York: Prentice Hall.

Moran, J. (1993, July). Ahhh, massage! *American Baby*, pp. 58-66.

Nakahata, A. (1992). Mastering Lamaze skills. *Lamaze 1992 Parents' Magazine*, pp. 38-44.

Noble, E. (1988). *Essential exercises for the childbearing year*. Boston: Houghton Mifflin.

Regnier, S. (1987). *Exercises for baby & me*. New York: Meadowbrook.

Schengel, J. (1991). Oh, your aching back. *Childbirth Annual Magazine*, pp. 25-26.

Schoen, S. (1992). *Fitness in pregnancy: Self-study guide*. Fairfax, VA: Author.

Simkin, P., Whalley, J., & Keppler, A. (1991). *Pregnancy, childbirth and the newborn: The complete guide*. New York: Meadowbrook.

Varrassi, G., Bazzano, C., & Edwards, W. (1989). Effects of physical activity on maternal plasma betaendorphin levels and perception of labor pain. *American Journal of Obstetrics and Gynecology*, **160**(3), 707-712.

Wells, C. (1991). *Women, sport, & performance: A physiological perspective*. Champaign, IL: Human Kinetics.

White, J. (1992, May). Exercising for two: What's safe for the active pregnant woman? *The Physician and Sportsmedicine*, pp. 179-186.

# Index